THE HE

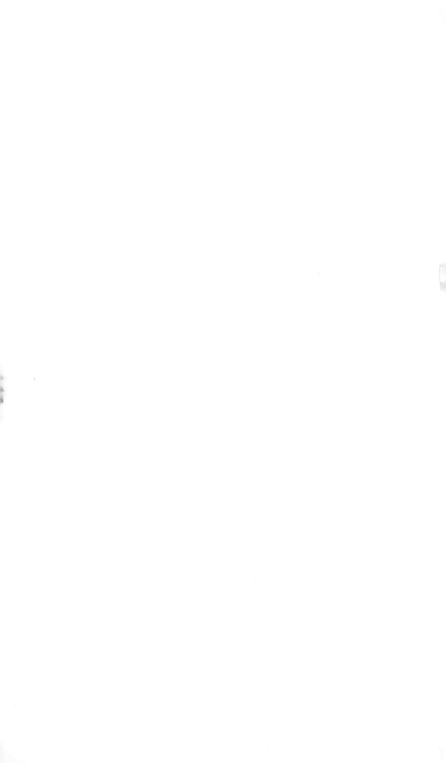

THE
HEALTH
FACTOR

ANNE MARSHALL

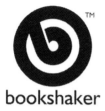

bookshaker

First Published in Great Britain 2010
by www.BookShaker.com

To my husband John, whose love sustains me.

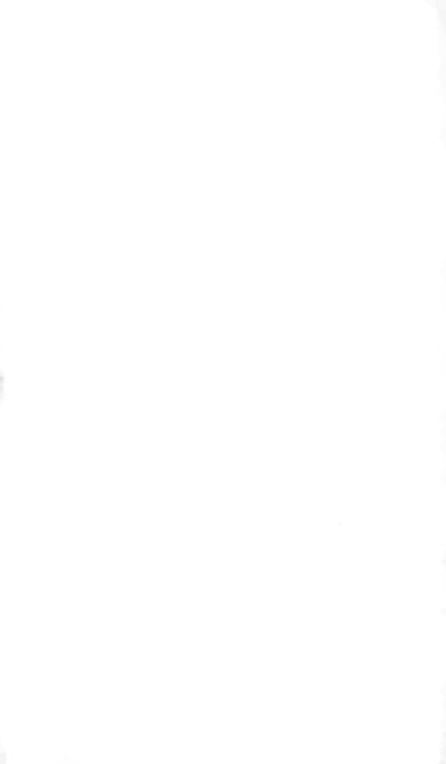

ACKNOWLEDGEMENTS

Amongst the many people I would like to thank for their help and influence in writing this book are my teachers and fellow practitioners whose wisdom and encouragement has served to guide me so well on my own coaching journey. My particular thanks go to Lynda Hudson for her companionship and honest insights and to Debbie Jenkins and Joe Gregory of Bookshaker, without whom this book would not have been possible.

Last but not least my heartfelt thanks go out to all my coaching clients who have inspired me and taught me so much over the years. Thank you for allowing me to grow and learn alongside you.

DISCLAIMER

ABOUT ANNE MARSHALL

Anne Marshall is a Clinical Hypnotherapist and Health Coach with an extensive background in conventional healthcare. She holds accreditation as a Master Certified Coach with the International Institute of Coaching and is well known both nationally and internationally as a speaker, seminar presenter, and personal coach.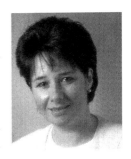

This book is based on her highly acclaimed Wellness Coaching Programme and as well as running a busy coaching practice Anne offers a wide range of seminars in the field of Health and Wellness Coaching. She is the author of many articles and training packages that have reached audiences across the globe.

Based in the heart of rural Devon where she lives with her husband John, Anne's aim is simply to help the people she works with to find and then maintain their very best level of health, wellbeing and fulfilment.

Learn more at *www.AnneLesleyMarshall.co.uk*

"I want to do with you what spring does with the cherry trees."
PABLO NERUDA CHILEAN POET, DIPLOMAT AND POLITICIAN

PRAISE

"Anne Marshall is efficacious on every level and incisive too. She brings genuine expertise, experience, encouragement and illumination. Ever generous with her help, we are lucky with this timely gift of her book."
Nicola James, BADipCMTh. University Mental Health and Wellbeing Team Leader, Chaplain and Writer

"I love this book. As I started to read, I found myself realising that it could have been written for me and I found that I was being irresistibly drawn to the idea of becoming my own health coach. Anne Marshall's style is warm and encouraging, she clearly writes from experience and has a natural authority which is reassuring and, at the same time, entices you towards a sense of vitality and inner wellness."
Lynda Hudson, Author of 'Scripts and Strategies in Hypnotherapy with Children' and 'More Scripts and Strategies in Hypnotherapy'

"Written in a clear and inspiring style, The Health Factor offers you a simple and highly accessible self–coaching programme. Throughout this book Anne Marshall shares with you the basic principles of NLP and coaching; and provides a structure within which you can develop the skills to become your own personal health coach."
George Houguez, D.Hyp., PDCHyp., PDCBHyp., MBSCH., The London College of Clinical Hypnosis, www.lcch.co.uk

"This book is not a 'read' it is Anne Marshall beside you every step of the way to a profound understanding of health; inspiring the desire for that health, the sound strategies and tools for achieving it and that glow of happiness and satisfaction that can make us role models for others."
Caroline Minto, www.thehenhouseblog.com

"This book's clear, engaging and warm style quickly draws the reader into feeling that Anne must know them! We all have small (or big) niggling worries about some aspect of our health and well-being and this book encourages us to invest in improvement. Anne is straight talking and helps us to decide how much of ourselves we will put into the process. The practical, clear and above all, gentle encouragement is sure to be a positive read for most of us and demystifies what coaching can do for our well being. Thank you, Anne."
Jane Watt, BA, CQSW, Life Coach, EFT practitioner,
www.branchingoutwards.com

"This book is a must read for all who value their personal health and wellbeing. None of us know the challenges that we are likely to face as we grow older and go through life, Anne makes it perfectly clear we do have a choice and maps out the way forward. I will be recommending this highly to friends, family, and business clients as it provides a positive alternative to fear, struggle, and just plain resignation. It is beautifully written in language that is easy to understand. The explanations and coaching exercises are thought provoking and life changing. This should be recommended reading for anyone training to be a coach, as health and wellbeing are fundamental to who we are and how we experience the world."
Liz Tyas-Peterson BSc., www.bluestarukservices.co.uk

"No-one knows the true value of their own health until they lose it! Therefore, what Anne has miraculously created with her book, is a hand-holding, intimate guide for those on the journey towards regaining their health and well-being and for those who are looking to take their health to the next level."
Carrie Eddins, www.chocolaterehab.com

"This book resonated with me. It is full of wonderful hints and tools to enable you to be more aware of your health and wellness. As a retired doctor who became a life coach I am more and more aware of how important the concepts described by Anne are to help us all lead a fuller and happier life."
Susan Kersley, www.thedoctorscoach.co.uk

"This is an excellent book covering all the main points in the quest for improved health. The importance of recognising negative self-talk and reframing unhelpful beliefs came across strongly and the client examples really helped to bring the book to life."
Deirdre Dee, www.deirdredee.com

"This is a practical book - to the point, with loads of variety, activity and alternatives. Established coaching and change models sit alongside original ideas, making this a work accessible for all."
David Miskimin, Co-Author 'The Coaching Parent',
www.thecoachingparent.com, Director, www.thedirectorscoach.com

"Anne Marshall's style is simple, yet profound, gentle, yet thought provoking. The Health Factor is packed with practical tools, I highly recommend you read it in order to make changes now!"
Annie Ashdown, Co-Host of Kyle's Academy (ITV 1),
www.selfconfidencecentre.com

"I highly recommend this book to all those who believe in being healthy. Anne Marshall is an excellent Health Coach. Her experience shows that she can guide you and your family towards better and healthy living. She is a fountain of knowledge in her discipline."
Salman Dossa, Youth Coach & Trainer, www.createyourdestiny.co.uk

CONTENTS

FOREWORD

When Anne Marshall mentioned she was thinking about writing a 'coaching and health' book, I was not the least bit surprised. In fact, I supported the idea wholeheartedly. You see, Anne is a long-time friend of mine, and a magnificent coach whom I have always admired. Her work in the field of coaching, especially health coaching, is unique and so far beyond what others would call 'cutting edge', I'm not sure there is a word to accurately express it. I have always believed Anne to be one of the most warm, caring, truly insightful people on the planet. She is that rare combination of warmth and intelligence. In Anne's presence, you know you are speaking with someone really special... someone determined to overcome every roadblock and make a real difference in the lives of others.

You would think these qualities would be enough to endear Anne to me, but wait... there is more.

I'm Gerard O'Donovan, founder of Noble-Manhattan Coaching, a European leader in the billion-dollar coaching industry. Since the inception of Noble-Manhattan Coaching in 1996 until today, my organization has trained more than 5000 coaches across the globe, in more than 26 countries. I think it is safe to say I know coaching talent when I see it. Anne Marshall has what it takes. She consistently reaches and exceeds the highest coaching standards, continually working to improve her fantastic coaching methods, always with an eye to helping others achieve greater health and happiness.

Throughout this book, Anne outlines step by step, proven coaching methods very near and dear to my own heart, and my own coaching beliefs; in particular, her discussions of false beliefs, the meaning of consequences, overcoming excuses, and using your own innate gifts to take control of your own health.

Of course, simply reading a book won't necessarily change longstanding habits and beliefs. Anne is highly aware of this. She knows there is more to wellbeing than physical change. That is why Anne Marshall will also help you make a 'conscious connection', creating meaningful goals that will teach you how to coach yourself to better health, for greater vitality and wellbeing for years to come.

And who doesn't want that?

Gerard O'Donovan

Founder of Noble Manhattan Coaching (www.noble-manhattan.com)
President of the IIC (International Institute of Coaching)

CHAPTER ONE

ARE YOU READY TO CHERISH YOUR HEALTH?

*"Cherish your health. If it is good, preserve it.
If it is unstable, improve it. If it is beyond
what you can improve, get help."*
GEORGE CARLIN, AMERICAN ACTOR AND AUTHOR 1937

It has been said that enjoying good mental, emotional and physical wellbeing is the very foundation of enjoying life at its best. Sadly though, most of us were never taught the life skills that we really need to make optimal wellbeing a practical reality.

In this book I would like to help change that. I will show you how you can take some simple but effective steps to coach yourself to better health, in short I will tempt you to have just a little more care and respect for yourself.

We have become used to a world of quick fixes and instant gratification and it's not unusual to find ourselves presented with a bewildering array of wellness guides, services and products, many of which offer us temporary fixes at best. It can be genuinely difficult to know which road to follow or which product or service might actually be of help.

Creating an improvement in your baseline level of wellness can be hard. Keeping that improvement can be even harder and yet you actually have a wealth of resources to help you, right within you. Resources that you probably don't even know about. Resources that will make the process of change much easier than you could ever have imagined.

As a health and wellness coach my role is to help you find and then use those resources, to energise your commitment to something better, to encourage you to take responsibility for your own wellbeing and in the process to take real and practical steps towards enjoying better health and greater wellness.

I'm not going to make it easy for you by giving you all the answers. I will be encouraging you to find your own answers and I will be showing you how in very simple, practical and sustainable ways. I will be assisting you through every step of the change process, from identifying the gap you wish to close, through to raising and sustaining the motivation you need to close it, all guided by a simple and easy to use model.

I also want to help you to raise your confidence in your own abilities to succeed and show you how to be clear about why you want to change as well as the reasons you haven't changed up until now.

If you are already familiar with the coaching process then you will probably recognise many of the ideas presented here. They are after all, nothing new, just tried and tested tools that can help you gain a vision of your better-self and then make that vision a reality.

I'll begin by asking you to raise your level of awareness of what's possible and then ask you to take responsibility for that learning by putting it into action. After all, we have all experienced, or will experience challenges to our health at some point in our lives. Some of those challenges we can do nothing about, perhaps we were born with them, or aged into them, or were unable to avoid them, or heal from them. But for most of us, most of the time, there remains a measurable gap between the level of health and wellness we currently have and our potential to attain it. Sometime that gap is easily visible from the outside and at other times it is more deeply hidden within us.

This is not a book about miracle cures. It's a book about enjoying your best potential, so that even if you live with a serious illness, or injury, my hope is that you will still find ways to enhance your wellness within the limitations of what can realistically be improved for you.

The tools and techniques I'm about to introduce you to do work. I see evidence of that everyday amongst my clients, but you need to use them, reading this book alone will do little for you, you must take action, otherwise it becomes like looking at a road map and magically expecting to arrive at your destination without making the effort to plan your route, or even get in the car. In other words without some focused commitment on your part your destination will just remain a daydream.

Change is seldom easy. It takes courage and being told by your doctor or even by friends and family that you should change often isn't enough to actually get you there. But health coaching has a secret ingredient to offer you and that is the encouragement to take a greater responsibility for yourself.

So as the pages of this book unfold I hope to be able to speak to that part of you that knows that it is possible to enjoy better health and to en-courage you to take what I hope will be the first of many steps towards greater wellness, whatever that means to you.

You can do it. I know you can and I'll be here beside you to help you on your way.

IT'S YOUR INVESTMENT

In this book I bring together the topics of health and coaching so that you can begin the process of coaching yourself to better health. In the first few chapters I'll be showing you how to make a conscious connection with what you value most about your health and then how to use this information to create some really useful and practical goals for yourself that can be used to guide and steer you on your path to greater vitality and wellbeing.

I'll show you how your inner beliefs and self talk can be harnessed to help you make the changes you desire so much easier to accomplish. Finally I'll be giving you lots of encouragement to complete the activities and to make all of this material as grounded and practical as possible.

This is a book about change and about enjoying something altogether better for yourself. It's not just about making physical changes such as losing weight, or changing a habit; enhancing your health can also be about adapting to a different lifestyle after an injury, major surgery, prolonged stress, chronic illness or even a bereavement. Improvement is always possible, the question is, are you willing to do both the inner and the outer work necessary to achieve the changes you dream about?

To help you think about this a little more deeply consider how fit and healthy you would like to be when you are in your seventies and eighties? What will you look like? What activities will you still be able to enjoy? If you are already over eighty, how about when you are in your nineties?

It can also be very revealing to ask the people closest to you what they think of you. If you are brave enough to hear some constructive feedback about yourself consider asking either your partner, or closest friends, what in their opinion would bring you better health. Ask them to make their answers as positive and constructive as possible.

HOW TO GET THE MOST FROM THIS BOOK

- **Set yourself some scheduled self-coaching time each week**. Make a date with yourself in your diary if you need to and make sure that the people around you understand that you don't want to be disturbed for a while.

- **Take it one step at a time.** Remember baby steps are fine, just as long as you continue to make progress.

- **Practice.** In each chapter I'll be offering you some tips and short exercises, so that by the time you have finished this book you will have a clear direction to follow and a good idea of how to continue to coach yourself.

- **Make use of the free website resources** that you will find at **www.Coach-Yourself.co.uk** to help keep you on track on a daily basis.

- **Find a trusted friend, or co-coach** to work with to discuss ideas, to brainstorm possibilities, or get support to achieve your goals.

MAKING USE OF THE ACTIVITIES

The exercises and activities suggested in this book aren't new, or special. In fact they are the commonly practiced, everyday tools of coaches everywhere. What is special however is how you choose to use them. I hope that some of these exercises will become trusted and familiar friends to you, whilst the remainder will also be able to prove their worth by teaching you something interesting about yourself. One thing is for sure, they will be of no value to you at all unless you actually use them.

All of the exercises are designed to get you thinking, to help you take action and to follow through on achieving really worthwhile results. Let them be a prompt for you to take better care of yourself. Of course, you don't have to complete any of them. There is no one to judge you and there are no qualifications to be gained, just the plain satisfaction of knowing you have achieved something rather special.

So do yourself the honour of completing as many of these activities as you can, make notes in the margins if you want to, or better still buy yourself a good quality notebook to act as your log book or journal so that you can take full advantage of what this book has to offer.

If you feel that you already have perfect health then good for you, perhaps you will be able to draw inspiration from some of the ideas here that will help you to protect that level of vitality and wellbeing that you now enjoy. If on the other hand you are simply not willing to change because you are too lazy to make the effort, or fearful of the life changes that might result from better health, then be honest about that and take responsibility for your decision.

Whatever your level of interest and commitment I hope that these ideas will help to inspire you, even by just a little, to take your first steps on the path to better health.

WRITING IT OUT

In many of the activities I've suggested I will be encouraging you to put pen to paper to help you recognise your thoughts and feelings more clearly. Some people feel that making written notes is not necessary and that they can make all the changes they need without completing the written exercises. In fact writing out your thoughts has tremendous value. It allows you to examine your actions and beliefs with an open heart and gives you a very practical way of getting information from the 'back of your mind' or the unconscious mind (where it is fairly useless to you), into your conscious awareness where it can be used. Many people are surprised at the quality of the information that can come through in this way.

At first completing these exercises may seem daunting and difficult because most of us are not used to expressing our innermost feelings, far less actually writing them down, but in my experience those people who don't take the time to complete the exercises achieve significantly less than those who do.

When you commit your goals to paper, especially when you actually write down a date for completion, you are in effect establishing a 'contract' with yourself and this can be a very powerful tool to keep you on track. I want to encourage you to have a go at all of the activities in this book even if at first glance they don't seem to be relevant to you. Do them anyway; you may well be surprised at what you discover about yourself.

So don't cheat on yourself.

Make the time and take the time to complete these exercises. I want you to get the best value possible from working with these ideas.

Remember change can occur very quickly, it is the not changing, that takes a long time.

CHAPTER TWO

CAN YOU REALLY COACH YOURSELF?

*"You cannot teach a man anything. You can
only help him discover it within himself."*
GALILEO GALILEI, ITALIAN PHILOSOPHER,
ASTRONOMER AND MATHEMATICIAN 1564 -1642

THE STORY OF COACHING

As this book is all about using the skills of coaching to help you help yourself to better health, it seems right to begin by taking a look back through time to the origins of coaching as a reminder of what it really means to us today.

In fact you may be surprised to learn that the story of coaching has its beginnings with an old Hungarian cart! Rumour has it that our present day use of the word 'coach' originated many years ago in the Hungarian village of Kocs, where fine quality carts and carriages were built to carry people between the towns with as much ease and comfort as possible.

Eventually the reputation of these fine carriages spread throughout Europe and with time the English word 'coach' came into use. So how does the original Hungarian word for a horse drawn carriage apply to the

9

modern day concept of a professional coach? One idea is that the more wealthy and privileged people of the day would have their companions read to them on long coach trips, or that a private tutor would use long journey times to read aloud to the children, and so the term to be 'coached' was born. Or so the story goes.

One thing is for sure, a coach, just like a traditional carriage is a means of transporting a valued person (that's you) from where they are to where they want to be with as much speed, ease and comfort as possible.

WHAT A PROFESSIONAL COACH SHOULD DO FOR YOU

Being your own coach isn't necessarily for everyone. It takes time and energy to make improvements in your overall wellbeing and occasionally it can be really helpful to have the assistance of a professional coach whilst you create the enthusiasm and motivation needed to achieve your goals or find a new balance in your life. Just in case this applies to you, or someone you know, I'd like to give you an idea of what a well trained coach should and shouldn't be doing for you.

Firstly they need to have undergone a thorough training and be properly accredited and insured and in my opinion they should also do the following:

1. They should take every aspect of your wellbeing into consideration, rather than focusing on a particular part of you that needs to be 'fixed' or altered in some way. All parts of you are related and work together as a whole and it's important to take that into consideration.

2. They should hold you accountable for the changes you say that you want. As adults we are

supposed to be able to take responsibility for the things we say that we will do but in practice it's not always that easy. A coach will help by providing you with the motivation and structure to be successful and stay on track. Remember your coach may be qualified in other disciplines too but they are not there to prescribe for you, just to hold you accountable for the changes that you have given your commitment to and to give you the encouragement to find out for yourself what really works.

3. They should keep you focused on your solutions, not on a list of problems that are holding you back and they should meet you where you are, however 'bad' that place may seem to be and then help you move forward from there. The entire coaching process is about your success.

4. They should offer you a short free sample session to allow you time to ask any practical questions you may have and to sample their coaching style. This also allows your coach to judge if they can really help you. Coaching is a partnership and both parties need to be confident in the relationship.

5. They may offer you 'signposts' to further resources but should stop short of prescribing for you unless you are also specifically employing them to do so, in which case they should hold appropriate qualifications in that speciality too. To tell someone what to do can be quite dis-empowering compared with giving

them the understanding of where they can get that information and learn for themselves. This is unfortunately why some coaches have earned themselves the name 'The Broccoli Police'. A good coach will never impose their judgements or standards on you.

So for example, if you are really overweight, or drinking more alcohol than is good for you, it is far more empowering for you to find out for yourself what a healthy weight, or alcohol consumption is, rather than have someone else give you a target that you must achieve. All the research shows that when you take responsibility for yourself in this way, you are far more likely to succeed in achieving your goals. It's what your health coach should be encouraging you to do.

These are just a few of the many benefits that a coach can offer you but it's worth pointing out that there are also some things that they shouldn't be offering you too.

In my opinion the best coaching is always content free which means that health and wellness coaches don't prescribe or advise. If they do then they are being something else. Nutritionists, nurses and personal trainers are all beginning to incorporate elements of coaching into their professional roles but if your coach is giving you specific advice about the things you should or shouldn't be doing, then it may be worth checking on their professional qualifications to do so.

A coach should never, in my opinion, tell you what to do, or worse still try to sell you anything, yet you will find plenty of people who do just that. So I urge you to make sure that anyone you chose to work with is properly qualified and that if they also want to sell you anything, or prescribe for you, that they are additionally qualified to do so.

Of course it's fine to combine coaching with other services such as consulting, advising, training or mentoring. In fact that often works very well, but I also believe that it is important to be clear about what the practitioner's scope of professional practice is in each area, even if they do overlap at times.

So if you decide to look for a personal coach I would suggest that you are really looking for a partner to travel along with you on your journey, pointing out the occasional signpost along the way, rather than for a teacher who tells you which way to go.

YOU CAN BE YOUR OWN COACH TOO

Wellness can mean so many different things to different people, to one person it may mean achieving a goal that is physically measurable, to another it may mean the ability to manage well under pressure, or even to enjoy a greater inner contentment.

In my experience most people already have a very good idea of what they should do to become more healthy, after all we are constantly bombarded with recommendations for healthy living by the media but many people also give up along the way, or fail to even start because they don't know how to work through the change process. In learning to coach yourself you can overcome these challenges by learning a set of skills that will last you a lifetime, skills that will help you achieve new outcomes for yourself that you may not even have thought possible.

Are you ready to coach yourself? You can if you want to, it is entirely possible but it takes focused commitment and a strong desire to succeed.

Are you ready for that?

If your answer is no, then be honest about that and consider using the activities and suggestions in this book just to help raise your enthusiasm for something better. Or consider accepting a free sample session from a professional coach who can work with you one to one.

If your answer is yes, then all you have to do is turn the page and we will get going straight away.

CHAPTER THREE

KNOWING HOW WELL YOU ARE REALLY MATTERS

"To wish to be well is a part of becoming well."
SENECA, ROMAN PHILOSOPHER MID 1ST CENTURY AD

WHAT'S THE DIFFERENCE BETWEEN HEALTH AND WELLNESS?

Have you stopped to think recently what your health actually means to you?

It is often said that to be healthy is to be 'whole' (hence the term holistic), but what does that really mean? What are the parts that make up this whole?

To be really healthy and well means so much more than merely the absence of disease. At different times we speak about our physical health, social, mental, emotional and even our spiritual health, they are all important and they should all be taken into consideration if you really want to get the best out of coaching yourself. Yet amazingly if you look in any western medical textbook you will be lucky if you find a good definition of health, let alone wellness and that is because there is no working model for anything other than sickness. Most of us have come to assume that the absence of illness equals wellness. But does it?

It's easy to define health as simply the absence of disease but I think that is really a very shallow definition and I suspect that if you think about it you actually know lots of people who have no apparent illnesses but who are not living truly balanced or healthy lives either.

Even if you are reading this book because you have a particular physical health goal in mind, I believe it is important to consider all these other aspects of your wellbeing too, so that you become aware of how they all connect together and form an integrated whole. Your health is about so much more than your medical history and paying attention to all these different areas gives you your best chance of maintaining a positive balance, even in times of challenge.

So if good health embraces all this, what does wellness mean? Is it just another word for health or does it contain more meaning than that?

In our modern medical world there are more ways than you can imagine to assess and measure the parameters of your health but to my way of thinking wellness is a much more subjective experience. It involves far more than merely the avoidance of disease or an early death, important though that is.

To me enjoying wellness is about enhancing the quality, richness and vibrancy of life to its maximum potential. In other words whilst good health may be seen at one level as an absence of disease, having a high level of wellness also means being in the best state that is possible for you, it gives you a sense of connection and meaning in life and allows you to enjoy a vibrancy and vitality that is more than good health alone.

As you begin to think about what this might mean for you personally you will probably begin with some fairly universal standards such as maintaining a healthy weight, eating a sensible diet, avoiding harmful substances, taking regular exercise and so on, but really good health is also about maintaining a state of balance and a sense of connection to the world around you. The way in which we all seek to find and maintain this balance can vary tremendously.

You will find plenty of activities in this book that will challenge you to find your own interpretations and meaning for these words and it's important that you give yourself the time to think, because if you don't really know what good health means to you it will be much harder to make improvements to your wellbeing, or even to recognise that progress when it comes.

Although I can't know for sure what your own definition will be, I hope that you will agree with me that enjoying wellness is possible even if you live with a chronic illness, or disability, or are feeling the effects of aging. You are so much more than any of the medical conditions or labels that you happen to have.

ILLNESS AND WELLNESS; A CONTRADICTION IN TERMS?

A question I'm regularly asked is, "can I have an illness and be well in myself at the same time?" I believe that the answer to this is, "yes you can". You can still be diagnosed with an illness and have a mindset of wellness at the same time and I know of plenty of people who manage this very well.

One very special way I have had this proved to me recently is in coaching people who are at the end of their life. You may think that helping someone who is dying to keep their wellbeing in mind just isn't possible but in my experience it's not only possible but also tremendously important to prepare well for this final transition.

Even if you disagree with me about approaching death with a mindset of wellness, I hope that you will agree that if you already have some limitations on your health, or have been given a 'label' by a medical professional that you feel compromises you in some way, you can still pursue a wellness lifestyle. In other words I do not believe that your level of wellness needs to be restricted by your level of health.

HOW DOES COACHING HELP?

Being coached or coaching yourself requires one fundamental thing and that is that you take greater responsibility for yourself. Before you can do that you also have to become more aware of any gaps that need to be bridged between what you currently have and what you would like to have. It sounds very simple, and it is simple, but you need to have the focused desire to make it happen and that probably also means you need to value and care for yourself a bit more highly than you have up until now.

Let me share with you some of the more common reasons I have found that people turn to coaching. You will see that in most of these areas it is possible to achieve a great deal by becoming your own coach whilst in others it would probably be best to work alongside a professional for a while.

- To fulfil a lifestyle prescription.

- To address a specific health concern (with medical support).
- To enjoy improved stamina or zest for life.
- To release a specific fear or anxiety.
- To improve levels of self-esteem or confidence.
- To be supported with 'skilled companionship' whilst undergoing a challenging medical or surgical procedure.
- To be supported whilst working through a major life transition, such as loss of function, change of body image, bereavement, or terminal care.

What are the main benefits of coaching for you?

Coaching works by drawing your attention to the impact of your choices on your health and then by helping you to work through or release any barriers that may be standing in the way of your greater wellbeing. Whatever you want to change or achieve it is a process that helps give you the structure to bridge that gap that lies in front of you, so that it not only becomes safe to cross to the other side but potentially fun and easy too.

ACTIVITY: ASK YOURSELF IMPORTANT QUESTIONS

It can be very tempting sometimes to take our health for granted, and it is often not until something goes wrong that we are reminded of our mortality. So I would like to invite you to start doing what you can right now to take even better care of yourself. Don't wait until it is too late, or too difficult, you can make a start right now by asking yourself the following questions:

- What is your own definition of health and of wellness?

There is no right or wrong answer to this question and it may well be that you have never really stopped to ask yourself this question before, but the answer is important. Take a few moments to write down some key words or initial thoughts as you consider this question.

- Now consider, what it might mean for you to enjoy even greater health and wellbeing in your life. What would be different?
- What will you have regretted not doing to preserve your health at the end of your life?
- What changes could you begin to make now?

We will come back to this topic time and again throughout this book, so don't feel that you have to come up with all your answers straight away. Your initial thoughts are important though, so do make a note of them so that you can build on your own process of self discovery.

You have a right to be well and very often all it takes is to have enough care for yourself to make the healthiest choices possible moment by moment. Sound's easy doesn't it? But the truth is that valuing yourself enough to always make the best choices can often be challenging in the extreme. It's why working with a health coach, or learning to coach yourself, can be the difference that ultimately make the difference.

CHAPTER FOUR

YOUR POTENTIAL AWAITS YOU

*"Most people don't need advice.
They just need support and discipline in
doing what they already know works."*
MARIANNE WILLIAMSON, AMERICAN AUTHOR AND LECTURER 1952

EN-VISIONING THE BEST FOR YOURSELF

One of the most important things I can do for you in this book is to encourage you to develop a better vision of your future health. Creating a mental picture of yourself enjoying a high level of wellness is an essential part of the coaching process because it helps you to connect your personal values to the importance of achieving a healthier life. It helps to connect you to what you will feel like and look like with your ideal level of health. Most of us spend more time planning our annual vacation than we do planning to improve the level of wellness that we enjoy every day but in coaching yourself you will begin to change that by focusing your attention very clearly on your best potential.

ACTIVITY: MAGICALLY TRANSCEND TIME & SPACE WITH A WELLNESS VISION

Just imagine for a moment that you could somehow magically transcend time and space and that, within reason, all the obstacles that at present stand between you and your ideal state of health could just disappear. In your imagination, spend a few moments already enjoying your best level of health.

What would better health look like and sound like, how would you feel different in your body? Would you be able to move more easily, sleep better, breath more deeply? What would be different?

Now extend this image a little further and imagine that you could actually see yourself in a full length mirror. Would your body size or shape have changed? Would you stand differently, be more relaxed, or even smile more?

How will other people notice that you are healthier? Will you be doing different things?

Close your eyes if you would like to and let this picture of your future self come to life.

Take a few moments to enjoy this daydream. Use all of your senses to make it as real and as vivid as you can, so that it can help pull you forward towards greater wellness. Then give yourself a couple of minutes to write about what you discovered.

Ideally your wellness vision should stir up some enthusiasm in you. It should represent a way of life for you that you would be really pleased and proud to achieve. As you begin to think about this, consider what new aspects of your wellbeing you would like to enjoy in the future. Things that are realistically achievable but that you don't have right now.

Use all of your senses to create a vivid picture of how your life will be different at the end of this coaching process. How will you know that you have improved your health? What specifically will have changed?

Throughout this book you will hear me talk a lot about raising your awareness and then taking a greater responsibility for your health, after all these are the key components of being able to coach yourself. So where better to start using these skills than in developing an inspiring vision for yourself.

This is an important step because before you can really make important changes you must be able to envision what you are working towards and really desire it to happen. Your goal must be your own and not just a lifestyle prescription that has been given to you.

ACTIVITY: LOOKING INTO THE FUTURE

What is the best state of health that you can picture for yourself in six months time? In one year from now? In five years from now?

Up until now what have been the main obstacles that have prevented you from achieving this?

What resources, internal or external could you call upon to help you move beyond these challenges?

ACTIVITY: DEVELOP YOUR WHEEL OF WELLNESS

This exercise is based on the Wheel of Life exercise as described by Whitworth in his book *Co-Active Coaching* (1998). It's an excellent exercise, much loved by coaches everywhere because it gives you a very easy way to see where the gaps are in your wellbeing compared to your potential for health.

In this version I ask you to begin by rating your actual satisfaction with a variety of different aspects of wellbeing compared with what you know is possible for you and then to repeat the exercise again but this time measuring your willingness to change by closing the gap between what you have now and your potential for the future.

STEP 1: DRAW YOUR WHEEL

Take a plain sheet of paper, or start a new page in your journal, and draw a circle divided into eight equal sections to represent your wheel. Regarding the centre of the wheel as 0 and the outer edge as 10, rank your level of satisfaction with each aspect of life that affects your health by drawing a straight or curved line to create a new outer edge. What is that new shape like? If this were a real wheel would it represent a bumpy or a smooth ride?

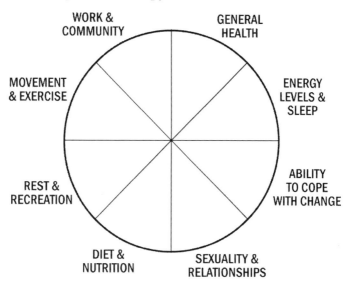

Jonathan's example:

Let me introduce you to Jonathan, a 42 year old sales executive and a self confessed workaholic who worked hard and played hard. He was apparently in the prime of health, his diet was impressively healthy, he enjoyed playing badminton and going for a run at the weekends and he was actively aware of the few minor health concerns that he had and was taking action to relieve them. But excessively high stress levels at work were really beginning to take their toll, he was no longer sleeping well and his relationship with his wife and children was deteriorating. For him the *Wheel of Wellness* exercise was a sobering wake up call. Have a look at how he scored his wellness in the areas of life that he felt were most relevant to him.

These are fairly typical ways to compartmentalize your health but I recommend that you chose your own labels to reflect what is most important to you.

- Exercise and movement = 8
- Diet and Nutrition = 10
- Sexuality and relationships = 8
- Ability to cope with change = 6
- Rest and recreation = 5
- General health = 6
- Work and the wider community = 3
- Energy levels and sleep = 4

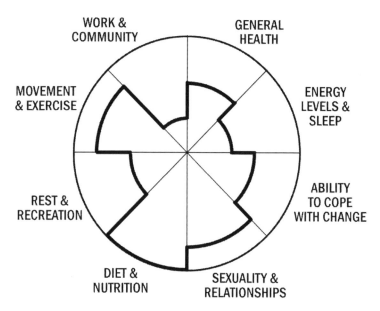

How did you get on with this?

Did you score ten in all areas? If you did well done, keep on doing whatever it is that you are doing. For most of us though there is room for improvement.

As a general rule if you find yourself scoring seven or less in a particular area then it may well be worthwhile taking a few moments to identify the areas you wish to work on or use as topics for your goals.

Sometimes, it can seem that there are too many aspects of our lives that could benefit from improvement and if that is the case for you, just step back and focus on the one area that you can change most easily.

STEP 2: DECIDE WHERE TO START

To help you find out what aspects of your wellness you would be willing to work on, I suggest that you take a different coloured pen, or draw a dotted line and for each segment of your wheel, consider whether you would actually be willing to make a change, again measuring your strength of commitment on a scale from 0 to 10.

If you are not ready to make a change or improvement in one area of your life, then just be honest about it and move on.

What do these two wheels look like? Are they similar or completely different?

In Jonathan's case he clearly had a good intention to make further improvements to the way he exercised and to pursue some general health concerns but these were areas that were relatively easy for him to work on. Improving his ability to rest, relax and spend more time on family relationships was much more challenging and this was reflected by his low intention scores in these areas. Have a look at how he rated his intention to improve his wellbeing:

- Exercise and movement = 10
- Diet and Nutrition = 10
- Sexuality and relationships = 4
- Ability to cope with change = 7
- Rest and recreation = 3
- General health = 9
- Work and the wider community = 5
- Energy levels and sleep = 5

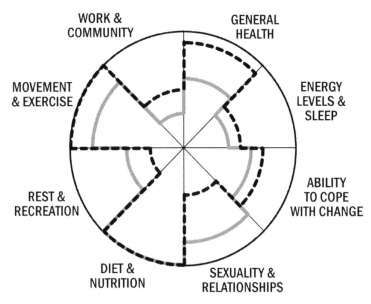

Wherever you find that you have given yourself a low 'wellness score' followed by a low 'intention score' you can be sure that these are the very areas that would most benefit from some coaching input. That said it is always a good idea to start with something a little less challenging, perhaps in an area where just a small amount of change will bring you really noticeable results.

STEP 3: CHOOSE A GOAL OR OUTCOME

Now pick one or two areas where you have identified a gap in your own wheel of wellness and start thinking about a goal, or outcome that you would be willing to work on.

For example, in Jonathan's case his initial goals were focused on improving his quality of sleep and protecting his off duty time for family activities.

28

TAKING RESPONSIBILITY FOR YOUR HEALTH

If you find that as you work with this material it sheds light on more serious health concerns for you, then please do go and get professional help. This is what health coaching is about, raising your awareness of what you most need and then taking responsibility for using that new information and this includes getting professional help from a qualified medical practitioner whenever it is needed.

Health coaching doesn't mean that you have to do everything all on your own, quite the opposite in fact. Nor does taking responsibility for your health mean that it is your fault if you have less than perfect wellbeing. Think of it this way, your response-ability is your ability to respond to the information you have, so if as you work through this book, you feel you need some skilled help along the way, then make getting that help into one of your goals.

For example, it is not unusual for the coaching process to flag up the need for specialist counselling. Sometimes when you shine the light of your attention on the gap between what you have and what you want, the apparent size of that gap can be overwhelming and for some people it can exaggerate feelings of low self esteem or even depression. So if this applies to you, know that this is a signal that you need to get some specialist help from a healthcare professional who can work with you one to one whilst you close that gap. It is by no means a sign of failure. Coaching is meant to direct you to the resources you need, both inner and outer, to help you move towards greater health.

WHAT IF YOU DON'T WANT TO IMPROVE YOUR HEALTH?

Curious as it may seem, there are times when the apparent advantages of remaining sick or injured can seem more appealing than getting well. It's a challenge that is well known to therapists and I mention it here, just in case it might apply to you.

For example remaining 'sick', or never completely healing from an injury (where medically this should be possible), can be a great way to avoid taking responsibility for yourself, for looking after your family or even for playing your part within the wider community. Sometimes when we can't say 'no' for ourselves we find a way of allowing our bodies to say 'no' for us. It's a well known way of avoiding situations and responsibilities by not being fit to participate.

As a health coach I come across this surprisingly often because the coaching process is essentially designed to fix your awareness firmly on your potential rather than on your limitations and just occasionally that can prove uncomfortable. In the end it is up to you what you chose to do with that awareness.

ACTIVITY: "I CAN'T DO THAT BECAUSE..."

If you were to raise your awareness of any reasons why you might not be willing to improve your health, what might come to mind?

Watch out for sentences that begin with the words, "I can't do that because..."

For example:

- I'll lose some or all of my financial benefits.
- I'll have to go back to work.
- I'll have to look after someone else.
- I'll lose some of the attention I currently enjoy.

What unspoken, unconscious agreements might you have made with yourself to stop you from improving your health?

These are hard questions that only you can answer, don't judge yourself, just be truthful, your wellbeing could well depend on it.

Now let's take what you have discovered about yourself and consider how to put it all into a realistic and workable action plan.

CHAPTER FIVE

IF YOU FAIL TO PLAN YOU PLAN TO FAIL

"Modern medicine is a wonderful thing, but there are two problems: people expect too much of it, and too little of themselves."
HIGH LEVEL WELLNESS: AN ALTERNATIVE TO DOCTORS, DRUGS AND DISEASE, DONALD B. ARDELL 1977

YOU ARE SO MUCH MORE THAN YOUR MEDICAL HISTORY

How you relate to your body's condition and how willing you are to embrace the possibility of improving your wellbeing will eventually have a great deal to do with the quality and richness of your life.

Modern medicine often encourages us to view our health as a set of fragmented measurements, such as our blood pressure or cholesterol levels. They are important of course but they are really just a tiny part of you. To pursue true wellness I believe that you need to look in the opposite direction, embracing all of your connections and relationships, including those with other people, the seasons, your wider community and so on. You are after all so much more than your medical history.

In this chapter I encourage you to write yourself an annual health plan, much like you would write a business plan in fact. It gives you a simple and practical overview of how you perceive your overall wellbeing and reminds you that good health means far more than trying to fit yourself within a standard set of measurements. Using an annual planner of some sort is also is a great way of giving yourself the practical structure you need to keep going and to ground your longer term vision. It gives you a continuous reminder of your own best standards.

WHY WRITE A HEALTH PLAN?

It has been suggested that almost everything we do begins with a well thought out plan and committing your good intentions to paper is an excellent way of setting goals that are realistic and appropriate for you and most important of all, measurable.

Writing out a health plan also helps you bring the ideas and intentions that may have been floating around in the back of your mind, into the front of your mind so you can be aware of them and then take responsibility for achieving them. It can help to show you just how much you are tolerating or putting up with in relation to your health. In fact many of these tolerations can actually be changed with just a little bit of forethought and effort and taking the time to write out your health plan is a great way of helping you spot the most productive places to place your effort.

Just like a business plan the purpose of a health and wellness plan is to help you identify what you will do and how you will do it. It will also help you to measure your progress and eventual success as well as giving you somewhere to record your most valuable resources and support structures. If you like you could also include a section on how you plan to reward yourself too.

Let me share this simple step by step guide with you, so that you can get started straight away. Use the template in the following pages or if you prefer, create your own.

ACTIVITY: PUTTING YOUR HEALTH PLAN TOGETHER

STEP 1: CHOSE HOW YOU WILL RECORD YOUR NOTES.

Choose either some good quality paper or create a new word document on your computer, so that you can eventually print out your plan and place it in your diary or somewhere prominent so that you can review it regularly.

STEP 2: CHOSE A HEADING FOR YOUR DOCUMENT

Head your document 'My Health Plan' or 'My Vision for Health' and if you think that you will want to share this information with anyone else such as your doctor or coach, then you might also like to include some general information about yourself such as your age, height, weight, current medical conditions or medications.

Allow yourself the time and space to write freely in this section to record what your ideal vision of health may be. Think about what your potential could be and ask yourself, "How healthy and vibrant am I willing to be?" Don't censor your answers. Just allow yourself to think freely at this stage.

STEP 3:SET ANNUAL GOALS

Take some time to look back at what you have written about your ideal vision of health and consider how this vision could be translated into goals that are actually realistic and achievable for you within the next twelve months. If it would be helpful you could also consider sharing your plan with your doctor or other health care provider who can guide and encourage you along the way.

STEP 4: SET QUARTERLY GOALS

Use this section to refine your vision even further so that you can see clearly which goals you would be willing to commit to over the next three months. It's useful at this stage to make sure your goals are 'SMART' and by this I mean that they are; specific, measurable, action based, realistic and set in time.

This is also a good time to consider the seasonal challenges that lie ahead of you. With all the wonders of modern living it can be very easy to ignore how your body naturally responds to each season. Whatever season is coming up for you next, consider what you could do to help yourself adapt to changes in climate, light levels, ease of getting around and so on. For example, perhaps you could eat more lightly in the summer, taking advantage of fresh local produce or even growing your own. Or in the winter maybe you could make an extra effort to take some exercise outdoors when the light levels are at their best. Whatever your seasonal variations are, consider how they might help or challenge your baseline level of health and how best you could respond to that.

STEP 5: PREPARE YOUR QUARTERLY ACTION PLAN FOR HEALTH

This is where you outline your strategies for success, and write down the specifics of how you are going to actually achieve some change, or deepen your wellness. What will you do and when exactly will you do it? For example, you might like to give yourself a wellness treatment such as a massage to help you unwind more deeply than usual, or perhaps chose an activity that will help you strengthen your connection to other people in your community by volunteering, or joining a group activity of some sort. These activities need not be expensive or even have any cost at all but they should help you to broaden the depth and scope of your wellness.

STEP 6: YOUR ADDITIONAL RESOURCES

Ask yourself what other resources if any do you need to accomplish these goals? Perhaps the advice or support of your doctor would be of help. Perhaps you need more information from a book, or the internet, to help you make a decision, or understand your health more fully. This is also a good place to make a note of what you know already works well for you, as this information can be surprisingly easy to overlook if you are striving to find solutions. It may be that you can achieve all you need on your own but it's always useful to consider building a support team around yourself for moments of uncertainty, or waning motivation.

STEP 7: SET YOUR KEY PERFORMANCE INDICATORS

Last but not least you need to record how exactly you will measure your progress. This last step is very grounding, it makes you take responsibility for the changes you are seeking and holds you to account. It also gives you a good reason to celebrate as you first reach and then reach beyond your chosen milestones.

Remember this is your own personal healthcare plan. You don't need to show it to anyone or discuss it openly unless you want to. Keep it in a safe place so that you can refer to it often and update it regularly. Oh, and one last thing, you may also want to create a log of your successes, even the small ones, so that you can celebrate and honour your efforts. Go ahead and give it a go, you may well be surprised at what you can achieve.

My Vision of Health

Annual Goals
WHAT I will accomplish this year

Quarterly Goals
WHAT I will accomplish in the next 3 months

Quarterly Action Plan for Health
My strategies for success – HOW I will do it

Additional Resources

Key Performance Indicators
How I will MEASURE my progress

Perhaps one of the most valuable aspects of mapping out your wellness plan is that you get to take charge of your health and express your individuality rather than just being judged by a standard set of clinical measurements. It can also help you to focus on prevention of future poor health by encouraging you to flag up the things you need to be doing regularly to stay in top form.

At the end of the day though a plan is just a plan, which means that it also needs to be flexible to meet your changing needs. It's a good idea to allow ample cross over between your shorter and longer term goals in case your priorities change.

GETTING THE MOST FROM YOUR DOCTOR

I often hear stories about people feeling that they have not got the best value from their doctor's visit and whilst it's fair to say that some of the reasons for this may be beyond your control, there are also a number of steps that you can take to help your visit be as empowering and informative as possible.

Here are some ideas for you to consider:

1. Take you health plan into your consultation with you and ask your doctor or healthcare practitioner to go over it with you. It need not take long but they may have some valuable contributions to make and it will give you a sense of teamwork and support that can be really precious. It also helps your care to be an ongoing process rather than something that just happens within appointment times.

2. Write down in advance of your visit the most important points that you want to get across. This could be your key symptoms or major concerns, or just some simple questions that you want to make sure that you remember to ask.

3. Ask for clarification if you are not sure what has been said to you. This is an amazingly common problem which can usually be resolved by simply asking your doctor to write down the names of any conditions, or drugs, or treatments that may relate to your care. At least then you have the ability to conduct some research on

your own, so that you are as well informed as possible. Never leave an appointment without being clear about what has been said to you.

4. Ask what you can do to help bring yourself back to health. Engage yourself as fully as possible and keep asking the next question. Ask, "what else can I do to help myself?" Then add this information to your health plan to keep you focused.

ACTIVITY: A LETTER FROM THE FUTURE

To help you think about what your health might be like or could be like a year from now, I've included this lovely exercise called 'A letter from the future'. This is a very simple, yet also a very challenging exercise and if you take the time to do it you will find yourself becoming much clearer about the aspects of your health that are of most importance to you.

Begin by choosing a date some months ahead or even a full year from now and spend a moment imagining what level of health and wellbeing you have achieved by that time. Now write yourself a letter from that point in the future telling your present self about all the positive changes, developments and achievements in your life. Be spontaneous and creative and complete this exercise without judgement.

For example, you could start by saying something like:

Dear...

Here I am one year ahead of you and I've got so many exciting things to tell you.... etc.

By writing a letter from your future self you are using the resources of your subconscious mind to help you tap into what's really important. It will prove to you that the goals you have written on your health plan are really worth something.

CHAPTER SIX

YOUR INNER COMPASS OF PASSIONS & VALUES

"When you are inspired by some great purpose, some extraordinary project, all of your thoughts break their bonds: your mind transcends limitations, your consciousness expands in every direction and you find yourself in a new, great, and wonderful world. Dormant forces, faculties and talents become alive and you discover yourself to be a greater person than you ever dreamed yourself to be."
PATANJALI, HINDU PHILOSOPHER 150 BC

PASSIONS AND PRINCIPLES

Did you know that discovering what your core values are in life and then honouring them is a fundamental key to your wellbeing and to living a stress free and healthy life?

Your values and most passionately held beliefs are what drive you forward, they are something you naturally feel drawn to and are quite different from your wants or needs, yet I have discovered in my practice over the years that in fact very few people really know what drives them on a day to day basis. Knowing what your core inner beliefs are gives you much more freedom to make healthy choices or plans that you can be confident will take you in the direction of increasing happiness. When you discover what you are most passionate about, you naturally raise your level of self-awareness, you get to understand what drives you and your important life decisions all become very much easier.

Whenever I give a talk on coaching or personal development I always like to ask the audience to put their hand up if they feel confident that they know what their most dearly held values are in life and the amazing thing is that each and every time I do this hardly anyone puts their hand up. Yet these are our most deeply held beliefs about ourselves, the core principles by which we live our lives and the standards by which we want to be known. They drive our life experience and yet we are hardly ever aware of what they actually are.

In fact I'm surprised at how often I find myself coaching people who have got to the top of their particular 'career ladder' only to find that they are leaning their 'ladder' up against a wall made of values and standards that dishonour them or that are in conflict with what they naturally value most. The result, not surprisingly, is stress and disharmony. One way to avoid this is to make sure that the 'wall' you chose to lean your own 'ladder' against is made up of the ideals and core beliefs that fill you with enthusiasm and passion for life.

Being really clear about what you value most and why is fundamental to maintaining a healthy outlook on life because your values act rather like your inner compass, guiding you so that you can experience greater balance, purpose and direction. If you lose this ability to make good decisions for yourself then you can all too easily end up allowing other people to make decisions for you, or find yourself taking on goals that aren't really yours. So it really is well worth just a little bit of time and effort to discover this essential information.

Even if you think you know what your values are take the time to evaluate them again because with the passage of time and changing circumstances, they can change, or alter the priority they hold for you.

ACTIVITY: DEFINING WHAT DRIVES YOU

Using these brief insights as a guide I'd like to suggest you take a moment to ask yourself, "what is really important to me in life?" Security, fairness, good health, love, whatever it is make a list of all your answers. Ideally you should come up with about 6 - 8 statements. Allow yourself to write freely, this is an important exercise and we will be coming back to it later on, so that you can refine your thoughts and put them into some sort of meaningful and practical perspective.

To be truly happy and healthy you need to be able to live in harmony with what you value most dearly and completing an exercise like this lets you see very clearly how much, or how little, you naturally appreciate your health.

Give yourself some time to consider the relative importance that each statement holds for you then ask, "which is the next most important to me?" Continue down the list in this way until all your statements have been numbered in their relative order of importance.

Next check that this sequence is really true for you by asking, "if I could have [statement 1]… but I couldn't have[statement 2] would that be alright?" If you are sure that your first choice is still more important than your second choice then you can be reassured that they are in the right order for you. If your answer is no, then re-number your statements in their revised order of importance until each has been checked for its correct sequence and you have a complete list of your life values and their relative order of importance.

Pay particular attention to any values which you initially identified as being low down on your list and which now move up to assume a much higher priority as this often signals an important area of your life which is currently unfulfilled and which may need to become the focus of some future goal setting.

Let me also offer a general word of warning here. No one finds this exercise easy. I didn't when I first tried it many years ago and I have found that a lot of people are hesitant at the thought of completing it. It can take quite a lot of courage to really look at what drives us forward in life and as you uncover what you are most passionate about, it brings with it the risk of highlighting the areas of your life that might currently be out of harmony with your most treasured beliefs and deeply held standards. So take courage and give it a go, what you discover about yourself may prove to be invaluable to your future health and happiness. Set aside some time today to make a start and then come back to this exercise in a few days' time to review your initial thoughts. This is definitely an exercise that you need to revisit a few times to get the best results.

RACHEL'S STORY

Rachel was a mother of two young children and a stay at home mum who had gradually started to take on more and more of the administrative tasks for her husband's business on top of maintaining the home and looking after the kids. She was washed out, exhausted and in her own words felt like a two dimensional cardboard cut-out of herself. Completing this exercise was a real struggle for Rachel because like many young mums she was so used to putting the family first that it was hard for her to even consider that she could have some values of her own.

At first all she could write at the top of the list was 'family life' but after a few days of thinking about it she began to add other values that appealed to her such as honesty, security and financial freedom. Low down on her list she also wrote the word 'creativity' and the more she thought about it, the more important that word seemed to be to her. On reflection she moved this value from number seven on her list up to number three. Recognising the importance this might have for her she started to include small activities into her working week that would help her express her need to be creative. She asked her husband to bring less work home and to help out a bit more with the children and with his support she was able to take up some sewing again, just for an hour or so a week.

In the end reflecting on her key passions and taking some positive steps to honour them made a really big difference. It helped her to feel more alive again.

WHAT HONOURS YOU?

To live your life with ease and passion your words must match your actions, which must match your beliefs and also your core values. Here are three good reasons why I think it is worth becoming more aware of what drives you. As you read through this list consider how these suggestions could apply to you too.

1. If you are clear about your standards it becomes much easier to identify the people, situations and things that don't honour you. When you next notice a person or situation that makes you uncomfortable or evokes 'negative' feelings, check to see if one of your core values is being violated in some way. Understanding this can help you conserve your energy from being expended in defending or protecting yourself.

2. Knowing what drives you also helps you identify and invite in those situations and things that you do want in your life. When you are clear about what matters to you most you can actively seek out the people, situations and things that support you. It helps put you in charge and gives you a sense of control.

3. Knowing your values allows you to be very clear about the standards you set for yourself as well as the boundaries you need to establish for the behaviour of others. If you think about it you will probably find that the behaviours which you find least acceptable are also those which violate your innermost beliefs in some way. Being clear about this allows you to easily establish healthy boundaries for yourself. It

doesn't mean that you are trying to change anyone; you just have added clarity about what is and is not acceptable to you.

ACTIVITY: HONOUR OR DISHONOUR?

Here is a short exercise that will begin to give you some insights by showing you what honours or dishonours you.

Firstly, think of two or three people who you really admire and would be happy to have as role models. Now write a brief list of the reasons why these people inspire you. What qualities do they have that you most admire?

Notice if there are any particular themes or qualities that they all share.

For example, when I did this exercise for myself recently I immediately thought of my favourite teacher. I hadn't realised up until then just why I liked her so much but apart from the excellent qualities of her teaching, she is probably one of the most generous people I know, someone who gives freely from a place of true inner abundance and who shows an extraordinary level of integrity in everything she does. I realised that one of the reasons I was so attracted to her work was that she was reflecting back to me qualities that I strongly admire.

Now, do the very opposite of this and think of a couple of people who you really don't respect. What don't you like about them? Be honest about this and for each of these things that you don't like, ask yourself which of your core values they are dishonouring?

Top of the list for me are people who lack integrity, because this is something I believe in very strongly and all that these people were doing when they acted without integrity was reflecting that back to me.

KEEPING IN HARMONY

To live your life with integrity and passion your words must match your actions, which must match your beliefs and also your most precious values. This is important because now that you have an idea of what it is that you are most passionate about you can take steps to honour those qualities by letting them shape your vision and goals.

Ask yourself, "what actions could I take to align my life even more closely with my most deeply held values and my strongest beliefs?"

The truth is that every single thing you do in life will either take you towards your values, or further away from them, and that includes your thoughts, ideas, beliefs and actions. With this information fixed firmly in the forefront of your mind you can become consciously aware of whether your actions and thoughts are magnetically pulling you towards your treasured goals, or blocking your path. At the end of the day when you set goals for yourself based on the values that drive you, you can also be confident that you will be heading in a direction that will bring you greater health and contentment.

ACTIVITY: REFLECT ON YOUR VALUES

Set aside a short period of time to look over your notes just to check that you have listed your values in their true order of importance for you. It's not uncommon for them to change from the initial priorities you gave them once you have had time to reflect, or after a major life change or illness, so it is often worth repeating this exercise from time to time.

Think about how you can bring these qualities to life on an everyday basis? For example, if you treasure your freedom highly, but work in a constricted and structured environment with little room for independent thinking then you are more likely to feel exhausted and stressed at the end of the day. So expressing your freedom in your spare time will become even more important to help you achieve a healthy work life balance. Being clear about what is most important to you also allows you to release goals that aren't really yours. Use what you have learnt here to help guide your goal setting as you work through this book.

CHAPTER SEVEN

WHY SETTING GOALS IS THE SMART THING TO DO

"Setting goals for significant accomplishments you want to achieve in your life, both personal and professional accomplishments, costs you nothing.

Failure to set them can cost you plenty. You are smack in the middle of the only life you are going to have. You can choose to succeed, or choose to drift; having goals makes the difference."

ALEC MACKENZIE, SPEAKER, AUTHOR AND CONSULTANT

DO YOU EVEN KNOW WHAT YOU WANT?

When your wishes turn into daydreams and then into active desires that are fuelled by passion and enthusiasm then you are ready to set some goals that will really work for you.

Goal setting is a powerful technique that allows you to expand your horizons and stretch your limits so that you can enjoy new or better things for yourself. They help to keep you focused, so that you can put your energy into doing the things that will give you real results as well as helping you to generate the persistence and determination that will guarantee your success.

Perhaps you have already noticed just how easy it is to say, "I know what I want," but when it comes down to the specifics what then? Do you really know enough about what you want to be able to recognise success when it comes?

Take the simple example of getting fit. I'm sure you have heard many people say, "I want to get a bit fitter," perhaps you have even said it yourself, but what does that really mean? What exactly do you expect to change and over what period of time? Failing to add specific details to a goal or new outcome is one of the biggest reasons for failure. It means your goals forever remain little more than a vague idea, unformulated, ungrounded and lacking in the specific details needed to give them the meaning and purpose to drive you forward.

Creating meaningful goals is central to the coaching process. Without them how will you know where you are going, how you will get there, or indeed be able to recognise when you have arrived? It is interesting isn't it, how many people spend fifty weeks a year 'planning' their two week holiday, yet give little or no thought to planning the quality of their lives.

One of the reasons that having an inspiring goal to work towards is so helpful is that it deliberately throws you out of balance by creating an image of excellence that is so much better than what you already have in reality and it is this conflict between what you imagine and what already exists that creates the drive and creativity necessary to pull you forward.

YOUR GOALS ARE IMPORTANT

So let's get down to some serious goal setting. After all it's just as important to have an honest and effective relationship with your own inner coach as it is with a professional coach and setting some valued and valuable goals for yourself is an essential step in the coaching process.

In the pages that follow you will find a number of exercises on goal setting that are designed to heighten your self-awareness so that you can act as your own coach in areas that are of importance to you. I recommend that you take your time with these activities and make a note of your findings in your wellness journal.

Take a moment to go back to those goals that you thought about when you completed the *Wheel of Wellness* exercise and use the check list below to make sure they are still appropriate and achievable.

- Make your goals realistic. If they are too ambitious you will be discouraged. If they are too easy, they will not stretch you enough.

- Make sure you are passionate about what you want to achieve. Believing in what you do creates focus, motivation, clarity and direction.

- Make sure your goals are your own, not someone else's expectation of you. A half-hearted effort is counter-productive and can end up being demoralising.

- Be clear why you want to change, what will your new goal give you that you don't have already?

- Create your own timeline to move forward. Aim to take at least one action step daily to reach your goal. So if you want a slimmer body then step on the scales today and decide exactly how much you want to change.

ACTIVITY: GOALS PAST AND PRESENT

GOALS FROM THE PAST

Before looking ahead to your new goals, it's worth taking a moment to look back to any goals that you may have discarded, or have left unfinished from your past. Consider:

- What goals from your past have you given up on?

- Are any of these goals still relevant to you today?

- Think back to about a decade ago. How did this younger version of you, envision your health being today? Was your vision of your future health very different from the actual quality of health that you have now?

GOALS FOR THE PRESENT

Review what you drew on your wheel of wellness and pick two or three areas where you rated the quality of your wellness at less than 7. What were those areas?

1.

2.

3.

Which of these areas would you be the most willing to work on?

Assuming you are going to be successful, what achievement would give you the most pleasure and the greatest return for your effort?

Now before doing anything else take a moment to check that this goal is in harmony with your values? For example, if you're tempted to use the words, I really should, ought, or must in relation to your goal, it is likely that this goal is more strongly influenced by the values of other people rather than your own. So consider how you could phrase your goal so that it inspires you and truly reflects an outcome that you believe is worthwhile.

Finally, remember that whilst your goals should always motivate you, there is also the danger that by placing your attention firmly on what you hope to enjoy in the future you can become distracted from enjoying the present. So keep this balance in mind and remember to celebrate your milestones of achievement along the way.

IT'S GOOD TO BE SMART

When it comes to coaching yourself knowing how to formulate goals that are 'SMART' will be a tremendous asset to you. Let me remind you what SMART stands for and as I do, think how you could rewrite your own goals using these guidelines.

S ~ SPECIFIC

It is important to be as specific as you can when you think about your goals. Being really precise about your final outcome is helpful because it lets you measure your progress more accurately whilst you are on your way. So ask yourself, what will you hear, see and feel when you have achieved success? How will you know that you have achieved this goal, what exactly will have changed?

M ~ MEASURABLE

How will you measure your success? For example, if you want to lose weight what will the scales have to read to let you know you have achieved your goal?

A ~ ACTION ORIENTATED AND ACHIEVABLE

If you don't take action it will never happen so it is essential that you take some action towards achieving your goal as soon as you can to help create the momentum you will need to carry you through.

R ~ REALISTIC

Ideally your goal should stretch you, but it shouldn't be so big that you feel daunted from even starting. Aim for a balance that is inspiring and stretching but not overwhelming.

T ~ TIMED

Setting yourself a time-frame for achievement is vital to help you stay on track. It also gives you a useful way of measuring your smaller achievements along the way. Use your diary or planner to record your target dates, even for the small milestones you will pass along the way. That way you can also be much more aware of your successes too and not just the distance you still have to travel.

ACTIVITY: YOUR MOST PASSIONATE GOAL

Taking all these factors into account, write down the goal you are most passionate about.

Don't just read these words and think about it, that won't do anything worthwhile for you at all. Go and get a pen and paper and actually write out your goal. Then write a date in your diary for completion and celebration. When you write down your goal in this way you are in effect establishing a contract with yourself to seriously do something about it. So please don't skip this step. Go and do it now.

Ideally you should review your most important goals at least daily. Write them out and put them somewhere where you will see them often, such as on the bathroom mirror or on a card in your wallet or purse.

So then, being clear about your values and establishing goals is important, but coaching is also about self-development and as you develop, so you will change and as you change so will your goals, which is why I would also recommend that you re-evaluate and if necessary re-write your goals at least once a month to be sure that you still really want them.

Nothing in life ever stands still, there is always movement either towards or away from your heart's desire, in fact every single thing you do in life either takes you towards your goals or further away from them, and that includes your thoughts, beliefs and actions. Once you realise this you can become much more aware of whether those actions and thoughts are magnetically pulling you towards your goals or simply getting in your way.

Enjoy your goal setting; it can be one of the most rewarding aspects of coaching yourself whatever area of your life you are focusing on. Keep your goals in the forefront of your mind and treat them like your constant companions, visit them daily and enjoy their guidance. That is what they are there for.

MARTHA'S STORY

Let me tell you how all this made a big difference to a lovely 62 year old lady called Martha who had recently been bereaved.

Following the death of her husband some 6 months earlier Martha had been finding it increasingly difficult to go out on her own or to spend time in the company of friends and family. Her sense of loss and loneliness were intense and she was slowly beginning to shut herself away from the world, largely because she had developed the beliefs that she couldn't make friends on her own and that it wasn't safe to go out without her husband. All this was made much worse as the initial support she had received began to fade away until the day came when she realised she needed to take some active steps to get out and about and make new connections before her health really suffered.

For Martha the coaching process involved a great deal of work on changing her negative self-talk, reshaping her beliefs and mentally rehearsing feelings of greater confidence. But alongside all this inner work she also needed to set some very practical goals.

When we first started to work together it was very hard for Martha to get beyond the words, "I can't," even though she really knew what she needed to do. What helped her most was breaking down her goals into tiny baby steps that were very easily achieved. For example, one of her goals was to meet a friend for a shopping trip in a town that she hadn't been to for a long time. Focusing on this goal was so overwhelming it quickly became more harmful than helpful but by breaking it down into tiny steps it became much more manageable. Her first step was to simply chat to her friend on the phone and arrange a place to meet that felt really safe to her. That done she planned her route in great detail, decided what she was going to wear in advance and so on. These were all tiny steps that added up to having the confidence and energy to actually go out and achieve her goal.

That shopping trip marked a turning point for Martha and she was soon able to turn her baby steps into confident strides.

I wanted to share this story with you in particular because some people think that goal setting always has to be about achieving massive change. It doesn't. Sometimes it's the baby steps that move us forward the most.

CHAPTER EIGHT

DO YOU HAVE WHAT IT TAKES TO COACH YOURSELF?

"Probably my best quality as a coach is that I ask a lot of challenging questions and let the person come up with the answers."
PHIL DIXON, OLYMPIC COACH

WHAT YOU SHOULD KNOW ABOUT COACHING MODELS

A key assumption in any type of coaching is that you are the expert when it comes to finding your own solutions. Of course you are, so that premise is contained within both of the models I'm going to tell you about, regardless of whether you are being coached by a professional, co-coaching, or coaching yourself. As you will probably have noticed by now, the coaching process is full of challenging questions and over the next few pages I'll be offering you a step by step guide through some of the most important of those questions. If you can allow yourself the time to answer them honestly you will find yourself transported along the path of transition with relative ease.

All models assume that you have the potential to overcome your own internal resistance or barriers to change but they also require you to have the courage and commitment to actually work with them, and not just read about them. A good model however should never constrain you but simply give you the necessary structure to make the process easier to follow. One of the first and best loved of all the coaching models is the GROW model that was originally used with great success in the athletics and sporting world.

GROW is an acronym standing for your **G**oal, your current **R**eality, your **O**ptions and finally your **W**ill to change. In this simple and practical model you are guided from your initial goal setting, through exploring the reality of where you are now in relation to those goals, exploring your options and finally confirming your commitment to take action. Here is a simple reminder of what those letters stand for:

- **G**oal
- **R**eality
- **O**ptions
- **W**ay forward / **W**ill

Although the GROW model is perhaps the best known model, from my perspective as a healthcare practitioner it lacks the element of safety which is so very important whenever you are embarking on health related goals. So I would also like to introduce you to a model of my own design; the OARS Health Coaching Model. I feel this model is more appropriate when it comes to making improvements to your health because it also asks you to consider if what you are doing is entirely safe and in the best interests of your long term wellbeing.

USING OARS TO MOVE FORWARD

Let me begin by telling you how the OARS model first came into being.

Like many coaches, I was reflecting on a recent call with a client and I just happened to be doing this whilst I was out in a rowing boat.

Now this particular client was a young man recovering from a motor bike accident and one of his key goals was to regain full mobility as quickly as possible. He hated hospitals, he hated being told that it would take months to heal and he had a burning desire to get back on his bike and start riding again as quickly as possible. For him the value of coaching was not in overcoming procrastination or staying focused but in having the skilled companionship of someone alongside him to share his progress, helping him mentally rehearse his recovery and above all encouraging him to make sure that his goals were safe and taking him in the direction of sustainable good health. There were many times in those conversations when he needed encouragement to seek out specialist advice to check on the safety of the speed at which he was pushing his recovery, and many times the advice he received was to be more gentle with himself, to have greater patience, or to exercise in different ways. There were times when that advice turned out to be very challenging indeed.

And I was reflecting on this as I was watching the oars of that rowing boat cut through the water pulling us further forward with every stroke and it occurred to me that this was an excellent metaphor for health coaching too.

Of course, if I had just looked at those oars they would have been useless to me. To be of any use at all I had to engage them with the water so that with the application of energy and effort they pulled me forward and it's just the same with the OARS model of coaching. You actually need to engage with it so that it can pull you forward.

So that is how the OARS model came to be born. I hope you find it as helpful as I do, but remember it's just a model, not a script.

THE OARS HEALTH COACHING MODEL

- **O**utcomes or objectives.
- **A**ction planning.
- **R**eality checking and locating resources.
- **S**afety check to ensure that your outcome, action planning and resources all lead in the direction of enhanced and sustainable health.

Here are some questions you might like to ask yourself at each stage of the process to help 'pull' yourself forward.

OUTCOMES AND OBJECTIVES

Firstly, choose the most important goal or outcome that you want to work on. Just pick a single topic to keep things simple for now. You can come back and repeat this process as many times as you need to for future outcomes until it is completely familiar to you, but for now I recommend you keep to one simple goal.

Having a specific and clear outcome is an essential starting point because it helps to give you direction and ground your vision by breaking it down into small and manageable steps.

Here are some questions you might like to ask yourself:

- What would you like to change or achieve?

Write your outcome in a simple sentence using positive words only to express what you want to achieve rather than what you want to avoid.

Imagine this outcome is already yours.

- What do you see, feel, hear, or do that tells you that you have achieved your goal? Be as specific as you can.

Check back to make sure that you have written your outcome in a form that is SMART. In other words it specific, measurable, action based, realistic and set in time?

- What might other people recognise in you, that proves you have been successful?

YOUR ACTION PLAN

This is where it all happens, it's where you decide which options will work best for you and it's where your commitment gets turned into real results.

- What now needs to happen to get you to that place of achievement?

- Consider what you could do to help yourself move forward. Think of as many creative options as you can.

- If you were to admit to yourself what the most important first steps were, what would they be?

- Now if you were to actually do these things, would they begin to move you forward in the right direction?

- What else could you do to put your ideas into action? Is there anything in particular that you either need to stop doing or start doing?

CHECKING FOR REALISTIC AND PRACTICAL RESOURCES

In this step you need to check that your action plan is actually realistic and achievable and then consider what practical inner or outer resources you could draw on to help you achieve it. So consider:

- What do you have now in relation to this outcome? What does the gap look like or feel like between what you already have and what you want or need in the future? How realistic is it to close that gap?

- What obstacles might be in the way of your success and what resources could you draw on to help yourself?

- Drawing on a wide range of resources, both inner and outer can make the process of change so much easier but most of us aren't used to asking for help. Where might you find the help and support you need to make achieving your outcome even easier? For example you could ask your doctor or nurse for advice, look for information in a book, or on the internet, join a support group, or perhaps speak to an expert.

- If you were to make yourself a list of all the resources both internal and external that you could draw on to help you move forward, who, or what, would be on that list?

KEEPING SAFE

Good health is incredibly precious so it's always worth considering if the people who are medically qualified to care for you would also be supportive of your plan, or would they urge caution about any aspect of it? Ask yourself:

- Do any of the goals or resources you have in mind compromise your health in any way?

Sharing your plan with someone who has the clinical qualifications to appreciate any risks you might be taking is not only a way of helping to keep yourself safe but also of gaining support for your plan too. So if you are not sure about the answers to these questions then I recommend asking someone who is medically qualified to advise you.

- Is your action plan fundamentally health enriching?

For example, do any of the resources you have in mind bring with them their own health concerns such as unbalanced diets, unknown 'medications', or stopping one bad habit only to replace it with another which can be just as damaging.

ACTIVITY: ASKING FOR HELP

Asking directly for what you need to support your success can be daunting sometimes, so it's worth giving this a little bit of forethought to help you find the right words to say. Here are some examples to get you thinking:

- "I'm doing really well on my new diet, please could you stop offering me chocolates?"

- "I want to cut back on how much alcohol I'm drinking, do you think you could help me by not expecting me to share a whole bottle of wine with you, I'd like to keep to just one glass this evening?"

Now think of some examples of your own:

- "Please could you help me by..."

CO-COACHING AND PROFESSIONAL COACHING

The golden key to coaching is creating an accountable partnership whether that is just with yourself, with a trusted friend or with someone who is professionally qualified to help you.

For really complex or highly charged emotional issues I strongly recommend that you find a professional health coach to work alongside you for a while. This needn't be a drawn out process but often the company of a skilled professional can prove invaluable in helping you gain momentum, or move through a challenging life transition. Of course you may just decide that you would enjoy the company of a skilled companion anyway, rather than going it alone, many people do and you might be one of them. But there is another option I'd like to tell you about that is becoming increasingly popular and that is co-coaching.

To co-coach effectively you need to find a partner who knows you well and who would also like to share a coaching relationship with you. Make sure you set some ground rules before you begin, such as maintaining complete confidentiality, equal sharing of time, listening without judgment and so on.

Check that you each know what the other wants to get out of the session. For example I often start with the question:

"How will you know if this coaching session has been a success, what needs to have happened, been achieved or understood, for you to really feel that it has been worthwhile?"

Then use either the OARS or GROW model to keep yourself on track making sure that you finish with an action plan that is realistic and acceptable and most important of all achievable in the time available between sessions.

To co-coach properly you need to be able to listen without interrupting, whilst paying complete attention to the strengths and inner resources of the person you are coaching so that you can encourage them to come up with their own solutions. It's also important that you secure real commitment for the action steps that have been agreed upon. And of course you should also expect your co-coach to be able to do the same for you.

ACTIVITY: CO-COACHING YOURSELF
Imagine that you are now the coach and you have been asked to work with a friend with exactly the same health challenges as yourself.

- What would your conversation be like as you take your friend through the OARS model? What new outcomes or achievements would they choose for themselves and what resources could you encourage them to draw on to help them achieve these goals?
- Now, what if this friend were really you?
- What is it that you know you need to do now?

CHAPTER NINE

WATCH YOUR LANGUAGE: IT'S FAR MORE IMPORTANT THAN YOU THINK

"Your mind can only hold one thought at a time. Make it a positive and constructive one."
H. JACKSON BROWN, JR, AMERICAN AUTHOR

INNER TALK AND OUTER REALITY

Your self-talk is constant. You are mentally talking to yourself all the time. In fact all day long you are giving yourself more advice, feedback, criticism and encouragement than anyone else ever could.

This mental chatter is often called your self-talk, or inner dialogue and it can have a direct bearing on your health and wellbeing, which is why taking charge of your inner talk is an important part of coaching yourself to better health.

For one thing, it has a direct bearing on your self-esteem, it also effects how you react to stress, your motivation levels and your outer performance, so taking the time to catch yourself saying self-deprecating things to, or about yourself, and then deliberately changing them into something more positive is one of the most important things you can do.

How often have you been aware of saying derogatory things about yourself either inwardly or out loud? Can you imagine speaking to your best friend like that? Probably not. Yet we all say things like, "I don't deserve," or, "I'm not good enough," on a regular basis and occasionally this can get out of balance leaving us feeling low in confidence and exhausted. Happily the reverse is also true; if your mental chatter is predominantly positive it can be a tremendous asset to you and it's one of the key steps in turning around your limiting self-beliefs and opening up new horizons.

Strangely enough when you catch yourself using negative self-talk, the first thing to do is to congratulate yourself for having managed to observe what you are doing. This is really important because without that observation you are powerless to change but with it you give yourself the gift of being able to chose again, and this time to chose something better in the form of words that reflect your true worth and potential.

Just consider for a moment how often you linger on past memories or images that are negative, deprecating, limiting or unhelpful. Most of us tend to let the patterns of our past colour our experiences in the present, yet the simple truth is this; if you spend time dwelling on negative images of yourself, then before you know it you will begin to believe that these thoughts and images are actually true and your inner-talk becomes a self-fulfilling prophecy.

It is all too easy to programme yourself in this way without even realising what you are doing. Vivid repetition of these imaginings can easily trick you into believing that this reduced and compromised version of yourself is who you really are. But it is not who you are and the good news is that there is no need to let the patterns of your past become your predictions for the future.

With just a little bit of effort you can reframe your past and make new choices so that you are no longer caught on the treadmill of negative thought patterns. The best news of all though is that this doesn't require hours of soul searching, just a willingness to go searching for new memories of those forgotten or ignored truths about yourself which uphold the positive qualities that you do want.

If you allow yourself the time to improve your self-talk I think you will be very pleasantly surprised at the results. Whatever you go looking for, you will find and it really is up to you which memories you choose to emphasise and accept as your truth and which you want to reject.

Here is a simple formula that is well worth remembering:

IMAGINATION X VIVIDNESS = REALITY IN YOUR MIND

It's a curious fact but your subconscious mind does not know the difference between an actual experience and one that is vividly imagined. This means that an event need not occur in reality for you to register either a positive or negative reaction to it. In other words when you imagine something with great vividness using all of your senses it can seem very real in your mind. In fact one of the functions of your subconscious mind is to ensure that you always act in accordance with your self-image which is why focusing on positive self-talk is one of the most important self-coaching skills you can have. After all no one can put you down unless you agree.

To stop thinking about your limitations, or stop running yourself down can be a challenging task, especially at first. Fortunately there are plenty of simple ways you can begin to make these changes and you'll hear me come back to this time and again throughout this book. The key is that you must be willing to practice and ultimately you must be willing to change.

For now I suggest that you aim to gently become more aware of the negative or unhelpful things you say to or about yourself and the next time you catch yourself being negative, make a deliberate effort to change those words to something kinder and more positive.

If you find this too difficult to do on the spot, then try doing something practical which requires your external attention for a while, preferably something that is fun and enjoyable that will help you to break that unhelpful thinking pattern as quickly as possible. Take a brisk walk for a few minutes, hum a tune, do the washing up, do anything that is easy and gets your attention out onto something practical. Then chose to say something kind and positive to yourself, however mechanical that may feel. Don't worry if you don't believe it, if this is a deeply ingrained habit for you, it is unlikely that you will be able to change these patterns overnight. But change they will with gentle and consistent practice. So don't give up, once you get into the habit of doing this you will soon find it becomes much easier to break patterns of negative thinking and you will save yourself a huge amount of mental energy too!

DON'T WORRY THIS WON'T HURT!

Even if you think that the essence of your self-talk is predominantly good and positive, the chances are that you still use a scattering of negative words in your everyday language. Words such as don't, can't, shouldn't and so on. They are negatives because they refer to you avoiding, or stopping doing something and we all use them in our everyday language. For example, "I can't stop thinking about those biscuits," or, "I'm really not going to have another cigarette today".

The trouble with saying these things is that your mind cannot process a 'negative' concept without first of all bringing into focus whatever is to be avoided. In other words your mind has got to call up an image of something before it can process the command to dismiss it.

Let me give you an example here. Have you ever been for a medical or dental treatment only to have the person caring for you say something like "don't worry, this won't hurt"?

What happened? Most likely you ended up thinking of the very thing you wanted to avoid, in this case how much it might hurt.

We always move towards what we picture most strongly in our minds regardless of whether it's in our best interest or not and this is really important to understand when it comes to making some positive changes to your wellbeing.

So when you use a 'negative' in your sentence such as can't or won't in actual fact all you are doing is focusing your attention on what you really want to avoid, such as that extra cigarette, or the biscuit tin. The trick here is to keep all your language positive and focus your attention completely on what you do want rather than on what you are trying to avoid.

What you say about yourself and to yourself will eventually become a self-fulfilling prophesy if you repeat it often enough. So it's worthwhile taking a few moments to scan your self-talk for any negative words or 'labels' that you may have given yourself, or been given in the past and then deliberately change them for something more positive. Simply by changing your habitual vocabulary you can quickly begin to change how you think and feel. If the words you are presently using to describe yourself dis-empower or dishonour you, then choose to change them right now for something new and more encouraging.

Your subconscious mind will go to work to create on your behalf exactly what you tell it to, so when old negative beliefs come up in your self-talk try breaking the pattern by saying something like, "although up until now I haven't [x], I now chose to [y]".

ACTIVITY: TALK TO YOURSELF
Consider the example below and then think about what your own examples might be.

Negative self-talk: I'll never be really fit.

Becomes: I haven't felt really fit up until now.

Becomes: I now choose... (be specific here about what exactly it is that you want)... and I believe it is possible.

New Belief: I am steadily increasing my fitness level all the time.

NOTICE WHAT YOU CRITICIZE YOURSELF FOR

When you hear yourself engage in some limiting or deprecating self-talk, ask yourself, "where is that message coming from?" Your answer may come in the form of a memory of something that you learnt as a child, or perhaps from strong influences that currently affect your adult life. The trick here is to recognise the 'voice' behind these limiting beliefs, so that you can consciously and deliberately dismiss it and deprive it of the energy of your continued attention.

Self-criticism can be exhausting and if it goes unchecked you can end up believing that your self-talk is really true for you and eventually end up depressing yourself.

If this is the case for you then it is a habit that is well worth turning around.

ACTIVITY: LET GO OF THE SELF-CRITIC

Spend some time today noticing how and when you criticise yourself and when you give yourself praise.

If you find it difficult to praise yourself then aim to say something good and kind about yourself at least half a dozen times a day for the next few weeks, to help build up your self-esteem and confidence.

The quality of your inner dialogues is really important and if you keep repeating self-defeating talk you will eventually defeat yourself. Coaching can help turn this situation around by enabling you to become more aware of any negative self-talk and then giving you the tools to change it.

CHAPTER TEN

YOUR BELIEFS ARE JUST THOUGHTS YOU KEEP THINKING

"We are like those well meaning people who visit a garden and believe in talking encouragingly to the blossoms when the real trick lies in talking to the roots. Down there is where the real work is done."

DUNCAN MCCOLL, 'THE MAGIC OF MIND POWER' 1988

THE FALSE BELIEFS THAT HOLD YOU BACK

We all have limiting thoughts about ourselves that stop us from improving our health and part of my purpose is to help you uncover those thoughts so that you can consciously decide if you would like to change them or not.

Often when we encounter resistance to what we think will make us happier or healthier it is because we have a limiting belief that is blocking us in some way.

What you believe represents the truth as you see it about yourself and whilst it is said that the truth can set you free it is also the case that some of the truths about ourselves are so imperfect that instead of freeing us they bind us.

Even though we act and live every day in accordance with what we think is true about ourselves most of us do not consciously decide what we are going to believe, instead we just accept our thought patterns that have built up over long periods of time and we rarely question them until we become so uncomfortable, or so limited, that we need to break free of them.

Bringing your unconscious thought patterns out into the open so that they can be seen for what they are is actually very easy. In a moment I'll be introducing you to a simple mind mapping exercise that you can use to uncover some of your more deeply held convictions that might be blocking you from better health. The exercise below will also give you a very good idea about what might be stopping you from achieving your goals. Do try it; you may discover some very interesting things about yourself.

ACTIVITY: FIND THE LIMITING BELIEFS

Consider some of your potential health goals, especially the ones you might be procrastinating about and then fill in the blanks in the following sentence:

When I... then I will be able to...

For example: When I'm no longer suffering from [x] then I will be able to [exercise regularly/eat more healthily/go out more/etc.]

Another example might go something like this, "when I'm more settled at home, then I'll be able to lose weight," or whatever is relevant for you.

Now look back at your answers. What did you write in the first blank space? The chances are that this reflects some very real and limiting thoughts that are keeping you from moving forward. Don't worry we all have them, the trick is to recognise that these beliefs are false, so that they can no longer compromise your quality of life.

Now look at what you wrote in the second blank space. What you wrote here usually indicates important and valuable activities you need to address or set as goals to achieve, whether or not you actually achieve what you wrote in the first space.

This is an excellent way of uncovering some of the more limiting beliefs that you may hold about your wellbeing. The question is would you be willing to sacrifice some of them in exchange for greater wellness?

WHAT DID YOU LEARN AS A CHILD?

As young children we all learned about ourselves from the behaviours and reactions of the adults around us. If you stop to think about this for a moment you will probably be surprised at how powerfully the medical history, ideas and experiences of those closest to you have directly affected your own beliefs about your health.

Occasionally our thoughts don't just hold us back, they can be potentially damaging too. For example, in my own case because I felt so close to my mother and had been told so many times how alike we were, I came to believe that I would end up suffering the same health challenges as she did too. Given that she died at quite an early age from a heart attack, this was clearly a limiting belief that I was better off without. Another less serious example might be, "if I go out in an icy cold wind I'll catch a cold." Not so serious you might say, but still not helpful either.

Here are some more common comments that I hear on a regular basis, use them to help you think about your own examples:

- I always get colds in the winter.
- I'm always slow to heal.
- I'm going to grow up just like my mother/ brother etc.
- Everybody suffers from [x] in our family.
- I don't deserve to be different/have more choice/be better than my parents.
- Everything needs to be perfectly in place before I begin.
- I don't have the strength to do this.
- I can't/don't know how to change.
- We are all like this in my family.
- I've tried all this in the past and it didn't work for me.

Sadly most people think these beliefs are also their truth, but they are not. They are just thoughts, not the real you and you are free to change them with just a little bit of effort.

ACTIVITY: WHERE LIMITING BELIEFS COME FROM

What ideas might you have picked up from the people closest to you about your own potential for good health?

MAPPING YOUR BELIEFS

We all act and live in accordance with our thoughts and self-images. They represent the truth as we see it about ourselves and your body is an excellent mirror for your inner templates. In fact there is now a wealth of good quality research proving that your body is constantly reacting to your thoughts and feelings. So although your beliefs may not be the whole story in terms of your health and well being, they will certainly be a part of the story, and that story is always worth uncovering, so that you can make changes if you want to.

As you may have already discovered from some of the other exercises, a great self-help technique is to turn anything that you want more intuitive or insightful information about, in this case potentially limiting thoughts, into a picture. This works so well because it helps you to create a bridge of awareness between the left and right sides of your brain so that your creativity can be accessed more easily.

Use the mind mapping exercise below to be really honest with yourself and you should end up with a good idea of some of the obstacles, be they real or imagined, that may be getting in the way of you reaching your goal.

ACTIVITY: "I DON'T DESERVE..."

Take a blank sheet of paper and draw a circle in the middle of the page. Inside this write a few key words to reflect a limiting idea about yourself that you would like to change. For example, if you are not quite sure that you deserve to achieve whatever your goal is, you could write, "I don't deserve" in the middle of the circle. Then mind map, brainstorm or simply write some notes around this central theme to uncover why you might be holding this belief.

Here is what a recent client wrote about why she thought that she didn't deserve to lose weight:

- I don't deserve to be as thin as my sister.
- I don't deserve to look and feel sexy.
- Being thin is for other people.
- If I lose weight I'll need to become more confident and I don't know how to do that.

Let yourself write freely, and you will probably be surprised at the number of thoughts you have that either slow down your progress or perhaps stop you from attempting to change at all.

Ideally this should be an exercise that you come back to more than once, especially as it can be quite challenging to complete. So be gentle and give yourself time to come back to your notes again at a later date. You will probably see some themes emerging which will give you a clue as to what might be holding you back and then you can decide if you want to change those thoughts and ideas into something altogether more helpful. You'll find lots of ways to do this later on in this book, but for now just be pleased with yourself for having uncovered some of the thought patterns that may be getting in your way of success.

We all have negative messages about what we are worth and what we deserve and these thoughts can often be severely limiting, or even harmful to our wellbeing but fortunately they can be changed, one thought at a time, simply by shining the light of our awareness onto some of our more habitual thinking patterns. This isn't always easy, or comfortable, but it is immensely worthwhile.

So be gentle and persistent and each time you come across a negative thought, know that it is just that, a thought that you have practiced thinking over and over again until you eventually believed it was true. Best of all know that you are not your thoughts and with just a little bit of effort you can begin to change them into beliefs that truly support and nourish you.

JACK'S STORY

Jack was a 47 year old musician who had recently been diagnosed as diabetic. This diagnosis was a huge shock to him and he was struggling to come to terms with the many adaptations he now needed to make to his lifestyle. By nature he was a tremendously creative and expressive person and he hated the apparent limitations and restrictions that were now being 'forced' upon him. Rebellion became his second name.

It soon became clear that Jack had a bad relationship with the medical team caring for him, he felt helpless and hated what he called the 'paternalistic approach' of the staff at the diabetic clinic.

It was only when we did some belief mapping together that the true reasons for his discontent began to emerge. Jack soon realised that much of his irritation at being treated this way stemmed from his early childhood, much of which was spent with his grandparents whilst his mother and father were working away. His memories of this time seemed to be dominated by being told what he could and couldn't do and of not being allowed to play freely. Soon enough, he came to believe that being told what to do in 'that paternalistic way' was always something to fight against. This was an interesting revelation for Jack because on the one hand he could see how this belief was causing him so much difficulty with his medical care but on the other hand he also realised how his need to express himself without constraint had also lead to a brilliant career as a composer.

Armed with these new insights Jack began to take charge of the situation. He spent hours researching his condition on the internet and within self-help groups and the next time he went to the clinic he took the lead by giving a really clear account of his progress and made his own suggestions for the next steps in his care. He came away from that appointment feeling as though he had regained some control and self-respect. He no longer felt powerless or as if the staff were talking down to him.

The staff hadn't changed of course, but Jack had.

CHAPTER ELEVEN

SO YOU THINK YOU ARE READY TO CHANGE?

"Change is a process, not an event."
JAMES PROCHASKA, AUTHOR OF 'CHANGING FOR GOOD' 1998

THE CHALLENGE OF CHANGE

The first and probably the biggest step this book asks of you is to recognise the need to make some changes to increase your wellbeing.

Very probably you have already taken this step and it may well be that you bought this book specifically to help you close a gap that you already know about and are willing to work on. On the other hand you may have been given a lifestyle prescription, or face a major transition in your life and simply not know how to go about achieving it.

A question I'm often asked is: "why is this so difficult?"

Surely if you know what you want, why you want it and how to get it, there's no problem? Well if only it were so easy.

The fact is that making improvements to your health can be difficult at times, especially when past attempts have been marked by negative experiences and failure.

Change is rarely just a one step process, if you have the energy, focus, enthusiasm and will power to make the improvements you need without resistance, then good for you, keep going.

More usually when you say, "I'm going to change," you move through a series of well recognised phases, starting with not being interested, perhaps even denying the need to improve at all, through exploring how to make the process as quick and easy as possible and then eventually actually doing something about it.

Having some understanding of these different phases is an important part of the coaching process because knowing where you are in the change process allows you to access the right techniques and resources to help you move forward to the next stage. It helps you overcome procrastination and fear of the unknown that are so often the cause of failure.

THE SIX STEPS

There are six well recognised stages of change, and if you would like to read more about them I recommend you read James Prochaska's excellent book '*Changing for Good*', but for now let me give you a short overview of each stage to help you recognise where you are in the process. They go something like this:

STAGE 1 - PRE-CONTEMPLATION

If you are reading this book because you are thinking about improving your health, or perhaps even been told that you need to change for the sake of your health, then you may well recognise yourself as being in this stage.

Until you recognise that you need to make an improvement or adapt to a new circumstance the chances are you will remain blissfully unaware that anything needs to be addressed, or even that a problem exists at all. In this stage your level of discomfort has not yet reached the point where the effort required to change has become worthwhile. It's a phase that is characterised by the words 'I can't' or 'I won't', then the day eventually comes when you realise that things are not going to get better unless you actually make them better.

This is the step I want you to pay most attention to because it reflects your inner acknowledgement that adjustments are needed, even though your conscious mind may still be resisting the process.

One of the greatest challenges of this stage is that when you put your attention on what needs to be done, often for the first time, it can actually make you feel worse, as you become daunted at the prospect of what lies ahead. This is a crucial point in the change process and if you get stuck at this stage you can end up feeling deflated and exhausted very quickly. Worse still you can end up going back to your old habits and thinking patterns having concluded yet again that 'it won't work' or that you can't do it. What you need to do is focus your attention on the probable consequences of not changing and then immediately start to put support structures in place to help you move through this phase as quickly as possible.

For example you could:

- Build up your knowledge about the risks and consequences of staying the same.

- Refer back to your list of values to help you generate leverage by increasing your desire for something better.

- Realise that your past does not have to equal your future.

Understand that it is entirely normal to feel ambivalence, reluctance and even fear about the prospect of making adjustments in your life. These are all very common emotions but they are not an excuse for ignoring your health.

STAGE 2 – CONTEMPLATION

In this stage you know that there is a problem and something needs to be done, but you don't necessarily know what to do about it yet. This is an information gathering stage where you are most likely to say to yourself, "I might change", but without making any form of real commitment. It can also seem like the low before the high as you place your awareness on all of the things that you want to be different, so it's essential that you don't let yourself become overwhelmed at this stage.

STAGE 3 – PREPARATION

At this point you have made the commitment to change but still have some preparation to do before you put those improvements into practice. There is hope on the horizon now and this stage is often characterised by the words "I intend".

STAGE 4 – ACTION

Success is now in sight. Your increased awareness, learning and preparations all help to raise your enthusiasm and motivation to succeed and your original level of discomfort starts to recede. At this point in the change process you are actually ready to say "I am..." One of the dangers here is that this stage can feel so encouraging that you might be tempted to stop before you have fully achieved your goal.

Don't stop. Keep your original goal up in the forefront of your mind and make sure that you keep focused on the specific and detailed criteria that will signal your true success.

STAGE 5 – MAINTENANCE

This stage is all about staying on track and moving forward. It's a case of "I still am..." and is characterised by the need for persistence until your new lifestyle overrides the old one.

STAGE 6 – RECYCLING OR RELAPSE

At this point in the cycle your new choices should be such an ingrained part of your life that they become automatic and go unnoticed. It's a time of celebration and perhaps also a time to raise the bar on your best achievements so far. It is also the time to consider what new goals you might have for yourself now.

Occasionally this point in the cycle can also be marked by relapse and if this is the case you will find yourself back at the beginning of the spiral of change yet again, contemplating and preparing for renewed effort. Don't beat up on yourself if this happens. Change can be difficult at times and it may well be that for some of your goals you need to take one step backwards in order to take two steps forward. But keep going.

ACTIVITY: WHERE ARE YOU?

Pick one of your key goals from your **Wheel of Wellness** and consider which stage of the change cycle you are currently in.

What could you do to help yourself move on to the next step of the process?

Here are a few examples to get you thinking:

- Use some of the self-help tools mentioned later on in this book such as affirmations or mental rehearsal to help bolster up your motivation for a better life.

- Consider what the consequences would be of not changing in one, five and even ten year's time. What might your health be like then if you don't take this opportunity now?

- Get some professional help from someone who is 100% supportive of you such as your doctor, nurse, nutritionist, personal trainer or coach.

What would be the single most practical and helpful thing you could do to help yourself follow through on your new choices and actually put them into practice?

YOUR CHAIN OF CONSEQUENCES

One of the consequences of health coaching is that it's not just the individual who is being coached who gets to benefit. Other family members and even work colleagues can often be inspired by your pursuit of a higher level of wellness. It's really a joy to see this happen but I need to issue a word of warning here. It's simply this, don't expect everyone else to get on board with you and share your enthusiasm. You may have decided to step out of your old comfort zone but if you happen to share that comfort zone with other people, especially close family members it can be very disturbing for them to suddenly have to adapt to your new way of doing things and this can cause great resentment at times. Once you are aware of this, it is usually possible to win them over, or to adapt your new practices so that the other people aren't affected.

ACTIVITY: DRAWING OUT YOUR CONSEQUENCES

Drawing out your chain of likely consequences is immensely valuable. Your potential results are made clearly visible and this makes it much easier for you to take responsibility for your choices, whatever they are.

There are two ways you can do this. Option one is to take some paper and draw a circle in the middle to represent the first link of your chain. Label this circle with some keywords that reflect the topic you are considering such as 'my weight' or 'confidence' or whatever it is that is of most concern to you. Alternatively you could draw a line down the page with spaces like rungs on a ladder up and down the line, again imagining that you are in your present situation in the middle of this line.

Beneath your central link or rung of the ladder, add some more links to reflect what will happen if you take no positive action. What will be the likely consequences for you? For example, if you want to lose weight but take no action you may end up feeling like a failure, not looking as you would wish, or increasing your health risks in later life. What would be the knock on consequences of this as the years roll on?

Now add some more links to the chain running in the opposite direction, to the top of the page, to reflect what would happen if you took some positive action to achieve your goal. What would your consequences be now? Perhaps a strengthened self-image, delight in looking at your new shape in the mirror, a better social life and so on. Think ahead a few years, what would be the future consequences to your overall health if you decided to take action today?

Here are some fairly typical comments to get you thinking.

Reasons why I don't want to change	Reasons why I am now ready to change
It will take too much time	I'm tired of putting up with this
We're all like this in my family	I don't like myself like this
I've always been like this	I don't want to lose my friends/ ability to work/ mobility etc.
If I do this, what else might I have to do?	I'm afraid of the consequences if I don't make this change
It will be uncomfortable / difficult	I don't want to take drugs/have surgery

When your chain of positive consequences becomes longer than your chain of negative consequences then you are really ready to take action. If it is the other way around then you will probably find that you had a low score when you mapped out your intention to succeed on the **Wheel of Wellness** exercise and you may need to do some more work to raise your level of motivation in this area to help you move forward.

Before moving on from this exercise, stop to think about how these consequences also relate to your most dearly held values and to what you think you want for yourself in the future. How big is this gap between what you value and want for yourself and the consequences of staying as you are?

The important point here is to know that no matter how big the gap is you can cross it. Improvement in your wellbeing, however small, is always possible.

OVERCOMING RELUCTANCE

It is said that whatever you resist persists. This is because it can take a lot of energy to actually resist doing what you know is really good for you.

Look back at what you drew on your **Wheel of Wellness**. What aspects of change were you ambivalent about, or even actively resisting?

If you are feeling ambivalent then you are probably feeling as though you are in a tug of war match between two opposing emotions that end up leaving you in a place of indecision and inaction. That is not a comfortable place to be. Of course it is entirely normal to experience ambivalence from time to time, in fact it can even be useful to give yourself that extra time for consideration, to really weigh up the pros and cons of what you are aiming for but it is not useful or healthy to stay in this place of indecision for very long.

ACTIVITY: ELIMINATE AMBIVALENCE

Consider which of your goals leave you feeling ambivalent. For each of these goals reflect for a moment on the pros and cons of staying the same rather than changing.

Before you can get past your own reluctance to take the difficult actions necessary for achievement you need to make sure that your desire for success is stronger than your reluctance to move forward. One way to do this is to make your future vision even bigger, brighter and more inspiring. For example don't just think about losing a few pounds, see yourself in fabulous new clothes, in new and exciting social situations, or shining with a new-found confidence. Create a vision for yourself that is so inspiring it actually pulls you forward towards your achievement rather than leaving you feeling as though you have been pushed around.

The people who are most successful at achieving great things usually have a compelling reason to do so. What is it that will compel you to work your way beyond reluctance?

Let me encourage you to make your dreams as big, exciting and undeniable as you can. Let yourself be inspired and enthused at the possibilities that lie ahead and you will soon find that you can swiftly move past any reluctance you may encounter.

CHAPTER TWELVE

DISCOVER YOUR TEMPTATIONS, HABITS AND COMMON EXCUSES

"Ninety-nine percent of the failures come from people who have the habit of making excuses."

GEORGE WASHINGTON, 1ST PRESIDENT OF THE UNITED STATES (1789-1797)

OVERCOMING TEMPTATION

If you have ever struggled to change a habit, overcome a temptation, or stop yourself from making weak excuses then you will already know just what a challenge this can be.

Habitual thoughts have a real physical presence in your brain too. The more often you repeat a thought about something the more hardwired it becomes in your brain, literally creating new neural pathways for your most common thoughts to run along. Fortunately it is also possible to literally re-write over any unhelpful old mental programs you have running, all it takes is focused attention and frequent repetition.

So the more often that you fire off a thought about something, the more hardwired it becomes in your brain too, until those thoughts and actions become well-established neural pathways and your habits are born.

This is one of the reasons why will power alone is seldom enough to bring about a sustainable change. Fortunately those neural pathways or routes of least resistance can be changed, and establishing new and healthy routines for yourself needn't be a struggle. But let's start by looking at what all this has to do with the role of temptation.

Facing temptation is entirely normal. Perhaps you have been tempted to raid the cake tin if you're on a diet, or to stay indoors curled up in front of the TV rather than taking some exercise outside if the weather happens to be bad.

One of the reasons that tempting thoughts can be so troublesome is that your beliefs and ideas tend to be experienced as real in direct proportion to the amount of attention you give to them. In other words, the more you dwell on a thought, the more powerful and real it will seem to you and the more control it will appear to have over you. This is why struggling with will power alone usually just leaves you feeling exhausted because in the very act of fighting off a tempting thought you are giving it the attention it needs to survive.

The key here is not to struggle at all but simply to release the tempting thought by placing your attention fully and completely onto something else. Over time and if left unattended your tempting thoughts can easily turn into your bad habits, so let me give you a few pointers that may help you break that cycle of repetition and give you the freedom to chose something new and more inspiring.

RAISING YOUR AWARENESS OF WHAT NEEDS TO BE CHANGED

By now you are probably fed up of hearing me tell you that the first step in the change process is to become consciously aware of what you need to do differently. It sounds so obvious doesn't it? Don't be fooled by the simplicity of this step. You cannot change what you are not consciously aware of, so without beating yourself up about all the unhealthy aspects of your life, or your critical self-talk, just allow yourself to become gently aware of your more common weaknesses that spoil your good efforts or get in the way of your achievements.

PREPARE YOURSELF FOR SUCCESS

This step is all about putting structures and practices in place to help yourself be successful, such as removing as many opportunities as you can for temptation to strike. So if you want to avoid raiding the cake tin last thing at night, then make sure that you don't buy any cake when you next go shopping. Give yourself the opportunity to do something different.

PRACTICE

Practice or repetition of the thoughts and habits that you do want is really important because this is what will eventually help you to re-write those pathways in your brain to reflect your new and healthy choices. One way you can help yourself is to use a thought stopping technique such as saying the word 'stop' or 'cancel' when a tempting thought or habit comes to mind. It is a very simple but highly effective technique that literally breaks up the pattern of your tempting thoughts, stopping them in their tracks and giving you a much better chance of consciously choosing to move on to other things.

Think about how else you could cut across some of your more unhealthy behaviours, to help yourself establish a new routine. For example, if you want to eat less you could try holding your fork or food only in your non dominant hand. The idea here is to deliberately do something that feels a little awkward or uncomfortable to help you stop eating without really being aware of what you are doing.

In the end much depends on how strongly you desire to change and how willing you are to practice. Remember that changing any habit has a lot to do with persistence. Some habits can be changed very quickly whilst others may take weeks or even months to change. Recent research shows us that on average we make a resolution approximately five times before we actually get around to doing anything different. So don't be average. Make yourself some new choices today, and start looking forward to that feeling of success.

Do yourself a favour and spend a few moments thinking creatively about how you can help support yourself. For example you could send regular and encouraging emails, voice messages or notes to yourself to remind you why you are making these changes in the first place.

Think about your own circumstances and consider what you could do to help support your success.

WHAT ARE YOUR EXCUSES?

Excuses are a great way of trying to hide behaviour that you are ashamed of and they are always harmful because they prevent you from succeeding. If you repeat your excuses often enough they will eventually become a habit and you will actually start to believe they are true. But they are not your truth, they are just inconvenient obstacles standing in your way for a while.

Here are just a few of the excuses I hear on a regular basis:

- I don't have time.
- I've tried that and it didn't work.
- I don't know how to.
- I'll do it when...
- It's really not that bad.
- I just don't have the will power.
- I don't think [x] would work for me anyway.
- [x] keeps me [y].
- It's not my fault.
- The damage to my health is already done, so it doesn't matter.

Don't delude yourself, none of these excuses are true, they are just a way we all use from time to time to absolve ourselves from taking action. They are all ways of relinquishing your responsibility to someone else, or to something else such as your parents, your genes, your hormones or whatever. It's much easier to make an excuse than to push through an old comfort zone.

When you make excuses it is often because you have a lack of structure around you to make the new decision easy and safe. Fear of failure or rejection are extremely common reasons for not even making the effort to begin to change so a good tip here is to break down any of the uncomfortable steps in front of you into even smaller chunks that you feel safe with.

Take the example of eating healthy meals. If it's too much to make the change to cooking with fresh ingredients all at once, you might be able to introduce just one fresh item of fruit or vegetables at a time whilst also giving yourself a structured plan of progress to attain your goal of cooking only with fresh foods in a safe and manageable way.

If you can't break your goal down into more manageable steps then look around for other ways that you can put some structures in place to help you succeed. So if for example, you goal is to get some exercise outdoors each day, say walking to work or the train station, but you hate being out in the wet and the cold, perhaps you could tell someone you are going to do it so that you feel honour bound to keep your word, or perhaps give yourself a healthy reward at the end of the week to celebrate your achievements. Think about this, what could you do to support yourself?

Have a go at the suggested activity below to help you become clearer about how you can change the worst of your unhealthy habits.

ACTIVITY: UNHEALTHY HABIT BUSTING
Make a note of two or three of your most unhealthy habits. It's OK to be completely honest about this. You don't need to show your answers to anyone else.

1.

2.

3.

Now write down two or three practical ways in which you could help yourself to change. Remember baby steps are fine, just as long as you keep going.

1.

2.

3.

Look back at those unhealthy habits you acknowledged a few moments ago. What excuses do you regularly give yourself for not changing?

For example, if your diet contains an unhealthy proportion of highly processed foods, your excuses for not changing may be that you were never really taught how to cook properly, or perhaps you don't feel that you have enough energy and enthusiasm to cook a meal from fresh ingredients when you get home from work.

Be as specific as you can. The more clearly you can identify why you stop yourself, the easier it will be to find a way to move forward.

My excuses:

1.

2.

3.

Now, how could you get round this difficulty, could you for example, prepare some meals in advance, or take an interest in a new cookery book? What could you do?

Would you be willing to do these things?

Coaches are used to hearing excuses all day long, so if you are going to be successful at coaching yourself you need to be honest about your own excuses too.

These strategies work because habits and temptations always rely on you feeding the thought with your attention to give it strength. Once you pay attention to the thought, the next thing you know is that you are deluding yourself that this thing, or behaviour is really not so bad after all, that you somehow deserve it, or that just this once it won't matter. Before you know it you have given in and that would be a great shame. So next time you feel overwhelmed by those unwanted repetitive thoughts consider these suggestions and tempt yourself to a change instead.

CHAPTER THIRTEEN

HOW NOT TO GIVE UP

"Believe and act as if it were impossible to fail."
CHARLES KETTERING, AMERICAN INVENTOR 1876-1958

HOW STRONG IS YOUR INTENTION TO SUCCEED?

Have you ever wondered why for some people making improvements to their wellbeing seems relatively easy and yet for others it can be a tremendous struggle?

One of the key factors here is your own belief in your ability to change as well as your enthusiasm to actually achieve the end result. In other words your intention to succeed is tremendously important.

What is your self-talk like when you consider some of the things you have identified as potential goals? Do you say, "I'm going to do this and nothing is going to stop me," or is it more like, "I'll give it a try if I can"? Which approach do you think would be the more likely to be successful?

If you fall into the category of just thinking you'll give these ideas a 'try' without holding any strong conviction that you will succeed then you are far more likely to find the change process a struggle.

This is why measuring your intention to succeed is really important. In metaphysical terms and even in terms of some of the latest research that is emerging from the field of quantum physics, it can be useful to consider your 'inner world' of thoughts as being just as real as your outer physical reality and so setting a clear intention can be a potent force in helping you to achieve your goals.

Let me give you an analogy here. Imagine the sun's rays shining through a magnifying glass that is constantly moving from spot to spot, the power of the sun's rays is diffuse and not at all effective. If on the other hand, the magnifying glass is held still and focused correctly, those same rays become highly concentrated and that diffused light suddenly becomes powerful enough to light a fire. And it's exactly the same with your thoughts.

So consider a goal that you currently have and ask yourself: "How strong is my intention to succeed?" Are you ready to do what it takes to ground your good ideas and turn them into reality? You might also like to look back to the **Wheel of Wellness** exercise and if you haven't already done so give yourself a score out of ten to measure the strength of your intention to be successful. If a score of 0 represents no commitment at all and a score of 10 represents total commitment so that nothing can stand in your way, what would you score right now for your most important goal?

As I often tell my coaching clients, a score of seven or less means you probably won't do it and if this is the case it might be worth asking yourself how much enthusiasm you really have for your goal.

Remember the word 'enthusiasm' comes from the Greek word *enthousiasmos*, which itself comes from the adjective entheos, meaning "having the god within". In other words it describes that inner passion and driving force that keeps you working towards your final goal.

On the other hand if you have a score of seven or more then you are well on your way to achieving what you want but it's still worth considering what it would take to raise your level of intention by just one more point.

Whatever your goals are in life, assessing your level of intention and enthusiasm can be a great way of checking if you are actually willing to commit to doing whatever it takes to be successful.

ACTIVITY: PAY ATTENTION TO INTENTION

Take a sheet of paper and divide it into two columns. Head up the left hand column "I want to:" and the one on the right "I intend to:" and then write down all the things you say you want to do, then the things you actually intend to do. Which column did you find it easier to write in?

Most people find that their list of intentions is very much shorter than their list of wants because for you to honestly say that you will do something your intention must be in alignment with your beliefs and values or you just won't have the enthusiasm to follow it through.

Let me put this another way by telling you the story of Emma's battle to stop smoking.

EMMA'S STORY

Emma was a bright twenty something business woman with a promising career ahead of her. She was also deeply in love with her boyfriend, desperately hoping he would propose to her. But there was a problem, she smoked heavily and he hated the smell of cigarettes. She was fed up of being nagged to stop smoking and one way and another their relationship was at an impasse. Fortunately Emma wasn't new to coaching, she had worked with a business coach in the past and we had already been working together for a few weeks by the time the issue of the cigarettes came up.

When I asked her how committed she actually was to giving up smoking she rated her intention at about two to three. She was full of resistance and resentment and even though she told me that she wanted to become a non-smoker, clearly her heart wasn't in it. Why? Because stopping smoking wasn't even her goal. It was a goal that her boyfriend wanted for her and not one that she had any real enthusiasm for herself. Once she realised this she was able to let go of the idea and focus on other matters that were really more important to her.

Some months later, Emma did stop smoking, but she did it for herself, not because someone else wanted her to.

WHAT IF THIS IS ALL TOO DIFFICULT?

One of the greatest challenges I find as a health coach is to be of help to someone who does not really want to change or who just isn't ready to change yet. Often these are the very same people for whom change is really important, perhaps even essential to their wellbeing.

I mention this because the chances are that at some point you will come across the same challenges too. After all, if you already had all the motivation and enthusiasm you needed to achieve your goals you probably wouldn't be reading this book.

Everyone struggles with a lack of enthusiasm from time to time and if this is true for you and you would like to do something about it, here are a few tips that you can use to take the first step towards reaching your goal.

Firstly get some genuine encouragement and unqualified support. A professional coach will naturally give you this, or you could consider co-coaching with a trusted friend who is willing to be fully in support of you. Sometimes good friends or relatives can play this role but watch out for them offering you advice through their own filter of opinions. Sometimes this can feel supportive but it can also make you feel as though it is their opinion that matters more than your goal. So be selective about who you ask for support and if you are not met with the right level of enthusiasm for your efforts, move on.

Secondly look out for a suitable role model, someone whose level of commitment you admire, or perhaps someone who has already made the sort of change you would like to make too and let them inspire you. The chances are that if they can do it, so can you.

Finally, by pretending that you already have the qualities of this thing in your life, you will find it much easier to go out and actually achieve those things in practice. A very practical way of doing this is to make sure that you always describe these activities in the present tense, not the future tense. So if for example your goal is to weigh less, it would be more helpful to say, "I am eating less," rather than saying, "I am going to eat less," because as far as your subconscious mind is concerned the future doesn't exist yet, so your intentions become meaningless. So keep your self-talk positive and in the present tense and you will notice a big difference in how you feel.

Procrastination is normal but there is always a balance to be kept between taking your time to reflect and then choosing the best course of action and getting on with it. Putting off something that you know should be done eventually becomes demoralising and exhausting and that's not good for you.

By now you will probably have gathered that the first step in moving forward is to become more consciously aware of what it is that you are procrastinating about, then you can decide to either drop that goal, or put some helpful structures in place to help you get on with it. But make sure you do one or the other.

Raising your motivation to achieve your goals is essential if you are to be successful. Without it you will experience resistance, procrastination and perhaps a sense of failure before you have really even begun. With motivation, your self-limitations will melt away and what might have seemed impossible to you before now merely becomes a realistic challenge.

In truth all change involves a loss of some sort. The loss of your favourite habit, the loss of your old comfort zone, or even of your most deeply held beliefs about yourself. So it is important to work through this material with compassion and gentleness, just as you would treat your best friend who was grieving over the loss of something special to them.

Keep going and very soon you will find that the pain of leaving behind what is old and familiar will be overtaken by the excitement of having something new and very worthwhile within your grasp.

With enthusiasm, passion and a strong intention you will find it much easier to achieve your goal, so it is essential that you continue to readjust your outcomes to make them more achievable, compelling and inspiring until you feel a genuine enthusiasm for them.

However just like the process of change, building up your level of motivation is a process, you can't just switch it on at will, it needs time to be nurtured and developed and the chances are you will need to work at it, so I have included a number of exercises in the pages that follow to help you do just that.

It is said that a journey of a thousand miles still has to begin with a single step, yet that first step really doesn't have to be the longest or even the most difficult.

Baby steps are fine, just as long as you keep taking them and they keep moving you in the right direction.

CHAPTER FOURTEEN

ACT AS IF

"There is no try, there is only do or not do."
YODA FROM THE EMPIRE STRIKES BACK

Over the years that I have been coaching I have come across a handful of helpful techniques that have proved their worth time and again and I have included a few of them here, just for interest in case you would like to use them too. They are not exactly 'coaching techniques' but they are all tools that will help you move forward and getting results is what this book is all about. I hope you find some of these suggestions interesting and useful and most of all I hope that they inspire you to go on your own search for the tips and techniques that will help you most.

SPEAKING WHAT YOU WANT INTO EXISTENCE

Did you know that listening to the sound of your own voice making suggestions for positive change is much more effective than the same words spoken by a stranger?

In fact when you record your affirmations or even just speak your goals out loud, your subconscious mind quickly recognises the authenticity and authority of your own voice and immediately goes to work on your behalf to help carry out your commands.

There are many ways of doing this. Some people are motivated enough to make up rhymes or songs and repeat them regularly throughout the day. But if like me, you think this sounds too much like hard work, then consider simpler options such as leaving a message on your voice mail to remind yourself about a positive quality, or thought for the day.

ACTIVITY: SPEAKING WHAT YOU WANT

Pick an activity that helps you speak what you want into existence. For example you could speak your affirmations out loud with authority and enthusiasm, or send yourself a voice message with some words of encouragement or congratulation for your recent achievements.

ANCHORING YOURSELF TO SUCCESS

Have you ever noticed how easy it is to form associations with things? We all do this naturally as our mind tries to make sense of our environment by looking for patterns and associations between things.

Perhaps a particularly striking piece of music reminds you of a time when you felt really good about yourself, or were doing something particularly exciting. Then again you may have had the experience of an unusual smell evoking memories of the more unpleasant kind, a lot of people carry these mental associations with the smells linked with hospitals for example. These natural associations of remembered stimuli and their associated responses serve to 'anchor' us to particular experiences and you can use this natural phenomenon to help move yourself into a more resourceful and confident state.

Very simply an anchor is an internal state which has been triggered by an external stimulus. You can create your own positive anchors by simply remembering a time in your past which also reminds you of how you would like to feel now.

ACTIVITY: SETTING AN ANCHOR

Start by thinking of the emotion you want to feel, for example if you wanted to feel more determined and focused then recall a memory from a time when you felt that way in the past. Let that memory be as vivid and clear as possible. Recall what is happening, see it in your imagination, feel what you are feeling, in other words, experience the event as if it was happening today remembering everything as clearly as you possibly can.

Let that memory build within you until it is really strong, then chose some way of physically anchoring that memory such as making a fist with your hand, or squeezing your hands together. Any simple and repeatable physical gesture will do. Then break away from that memory for a moment by doing something completely different before repeating the whole process again using a different but equally positive memory from the past. Do this with several positive memories until that anchor is good and strong. Then test your anchor to make sure it works by making that same physical gesture and notice how those positive memories naturally come to mind.

This is a great NLP (Neuro Linguistic Programming) technique that is simple, easy and practical to use, especially when you are feeling at your most vulnerable. Some people love it and use it regularly, others prefer different tools. Trying out different methods to increase your motivation and then learning what works best for you is all part of coaching yourself. Like most other techniques though, creating and then 'firing' your most positive anchors can take a little bit of practice, so be patient and have fun with this. You may well find that it turns out to be surprisingly useful.

PROMPT YOURSELF DAILY

There is no doubt about it; the people who are most successful are the ones who keep their goals firmly in the forefront of their minds. This is really a very easy thing to do and the results are usually well worth any initial effort it takes to set up your prompt.

Let me share a few suggestions here that recent clients have come up with, just to get you thinking:

- If you would like to take more exercise then keep your walking boots or running shoes by the front door so that they are easy to use. Better still actually put them on your feet when you get up in the morning, it will be much harder to curl up on the sofa with them on!

- Write yourself some supportive 'post it' notes with encouragement to keep going and put them in unusual places that you will come across during the day to remind yourself of your goal.

- Send yourself an encouraging email, especially if you are struggling to keep going. Send yourself lots of encouragement in any creative way that you can think of.

- Create a photo board, or collage reminding yourself of how you want to look or feel when you have achieved your goal.

- Join an online support group so that you can tap into the encouragement and ideas of other people who are going through a similar transition to you.

ACTIVITY: PROMPT YOURSELF
Now think of some ideas of your own.

AFFIRMING THE WELLNESS WITHIN
An affirmation is a positive statement created with the intention of enhancing your life in some way and if used properly they can be an invaluable tool in helping you to improve your wellbeing. They are not effective however if the rest of your day is spent thinking negative thoughts, or engaged in negative self-talk.

Many people don't even realise that their unconscious statements about themselves or 'self- talk' creates the bulk of their belief systems but in fact there is a direct link between your words and what you experience as real in the world around you. Many psychologists liken the subconscious mind to a computer, very literally creating the reality we program into it through the constant repetition of our inner talk. The current circumstances of our lives always reflects to some extent what we think, believe in and give our attention to. If you want to know what you are telling yourself over and over again then all you really need do is look around at the life you have already created.

Affirmations can be a great way of helping you stay focused on what's positive and good but let me also offer a word of caution here. It's simply this, sometimes, especially at times of low energy or vulnerability they can also have the opposite effect, in that they can put your attention very clearly on what you don't have yet and just trying to superficially overlay negative feelings with positive ones doesn't really work. In fact it can easily make you feel even worse as you reflect on the enormity of the gap ahead of you. To be of practical use you must to be able to connect with a fundamental belief that what you are affirming is at least possible for you.

If you find that creating affirmations just uncovers a whole heap of negative feelings about yourself such as, "I can't", "I'm not good enough", or "I'll never be able to" then take a step back and consider some other technique to help build up your belief in yourself, or strengthen your motivation. Alternatively try chunking down your positive statements until you believe that they are really possible. This may leave you feeling like the progress you are making is incredibly slow but that's alright. Slow progress is better than no progress and as your confidence in your own abilities grows, so you can begin to take slightly larger steps forward.

MAKING AFFIRMATIONS REALLY EFFECTIVE

You will find plenty of new age books full of affirmations but just reading your statement over and over again has been found to be only 10% effective at best and that really isn't good enough to make your effort worthwhile. On the other hand, psychologists have shown that if you can add vivid and detailed imagery to your statement, so that you can experience yourself enjoying your success with all of your senses, then over time this becomes up to 70% effective. The best news of all though, is that if you add the feelings of success to your imagery, even if you have to borrow the feelings of success from another time in your life, then with repetition your subconscious mind will accept what you are saying as real and it will become very much easier to enjoy the changes you desire in the real world too, not just in your imagination!

A SIMPLE SUMMARY TO REMIND YOU

- Reading only = **10**% effective
- Reading + Imagination = **70**% effective
- Reading + Imagination + Feeling = **100**% effective

This means that to be truly effective you must not only repeatedly visualise yourself being successful but you must also add the feeling or emotion of success to your image. If you can do this then your subconscious mind will be far more likely to accept what you are presenting to it as real. If you think about it the advertising industry also uses these same principles. The repetition of graphic visual imagery associated with a positive emotion can be used with great effect to sell you something and you can use these same principles to sell yourself the idea of some positive changes too.

I'll be saying much more about this as I introduce you to the amazing technique of mental rehearsal but creating some effective and positive statements that reflect the changes you want is an excellent first step.

Here are some tips you might find useful when it comes to putting your affirmations into practice:

- Firstly make sure you construct your statement using the present tense, as if you already have this quality or thing. Get personal and use your own name if you can so that your subconscious mind recognises the authority and authenticity of what you are saying. Most of all make sure that what you say is specific, accurate and measurable, just as you would if you were writing a SMART goal for yourself.

- If you can it is always a good idea to take the time to write your affirmations down. I know many people think this step is just a waste of time but in my experience it makes it much harder to deny this new truth about yourself if it is written down in front of you. It is also a way of highlighting your commitment to actually making a change.

- Connect with the positive emotion associated with your statement, or if that doesn't come easily for you then borrow the emotion from another time when the feelings of success were strong and then mentally associate those positive feelings with your words and images of success.

- Keep coming back to that new snapshot of yourself as often as you can throughout the day. This is also a great way of helping your self-talk to become more positive too. Repeating your positive statements regularly throughout the day is also important because it is known that on average it takes about 21 days of repetition to bring about real change and affirmations are a powerful tool for doing this.

- Finally, do a reality check from time to time to make sure that you do still want what your affirmation describes. If your original words no longer feel comfortable or congruent then change them for something more appropriate.

Nearly everyone I have worked with has been surprised at what a useful technique this turns out to be but as with everything else in this book, you will need to actually give it a go to find out for yourself.

EXAMPLES OF GENERAL AFFIRMATIONS FOR WELLNESS:
- I love the feeling of making progress.
- I enjoy the foods that keep me healthy.
- I choose thoughts that make me feel good.

ACTIVITY: CREATE SOME AFFIRMATIONS OF YOUR OWN:
Use the examples above to guide you, together with what you learnt from your **Wellness Wheel** to write some affirmations that will be useful and relevant to you on a day to day basis.

DON'T EVEN TRY
There will probably come a time as you are coaching yourself that your initial enthusiasm and motivation for change will be challenged by the task ahead of you.

You may even be left wondering just what happened to those genuine desires to do what you know will make you happier, healthier and more successful.

So let me offer you a good tip to help you get going. It's simply this. Stop trying!

Think about this for a moment, how often do you say to yourself "I'll try" (to achieve whatever it is). For example, you may say, "I'm going to try and stop smoking this year", or "I'm going to try and lose weight before my holidays". But what do you really mean when you say that you will 'try' to do something?

I always challenge my clients when I hear this word because more often than not what it really means is that they have already sub-consciously decided that they will not succeed.

Consider, what goals are you 'trying' to work towards in your life?

Now, what would happen if you replaced the word 'try' both in your inner self-talk and outer conversations with the word 'intend'.

Give it a go right now. What do you notice?

In general if you are willing to replace the word 'try' with 'intend' you will have a much greater chance of achieving your goal. The word intend implies that you are actually willing to be successful, whereas the word try holds little commitment.

If you find the word 'intend' too uncomfortable to use with sincerity, then be honest about that and think about revising your goals so that they are more realistic for you.

So there you have it, stop trying and start intending.

Now to help you a little further along on your journey of change, let me share a few more tips with you that you might just find useful.

SETTING YOURSELF UP FOR SUCCESS

Do what you can to set yourself up for success. By this I mean think about what structures you could put in place around yourself to make it a little bit easier to be successful. For example, if you are trying to change the habit of putting too much of the wrong kind of things in your mouth, such as cigarettes, food or alcohol, then find some way of interrupting this automatic action such as only touching those things with your non-dominant hand from now on. This will at least help you to break your unconscious responses so that you can chose consciously if you wish to go ahead. Be creative here and think of as many ways as you can of helping yourself succeed.

Next I recommend that you get some support, I can't emphasise enough how important this is. Going it alone can be really tough when you are breaking out of your comfort zone. Who do you have who could give you really unconditional and practical support?

Last but by no means least be kind to yourself. Remember that baby steps are fine. In fact taking small but positive steps on a regular basis can often be more productive than trying to take a big leap into the unknown. Steady and sustainable change is what you should aim for. Just like the story of the tortoise and the hare, there is much to be said for taking slow, steady and regular steps in the direction of your goal. That way the change you achieve is far more likely to be sustainable and you will soon be able to look back over your shoulder and be surprised at just how far you have come.

So be gentle, be realistic, look for ways to set yourself up for success and above all don't try!

ACT AS IF

CHAPTER FIFTEEN

WHAT YOUR INNER AWARENESS CAN DO FOR YOU

"Here is Edward Bear coming downstairs now, bump, bump, bump on the back of his head behind Christopher Robin. It is, as far as he knows the only way of coming down stairs, but sometimes he feels that there really is another way, if only he could stop bumping for a moment and think of it."

A.A. MILNE IN WINNIE - THE – POOH

I would like to introduce you to a few simple exercises that will help you create a bridge of awareness between your conscious mind and the incredible resources of your subconscious mind. Then most importantly I'll show you how to bring that information back into your awareness so that it can be used in the everyday practical world to help you make the best decisions possible for your health and wellbeing.

Avoid judging or analysing the intuitive insights you gain during these exercises. If you engage your logical mind to ask if the information makes sense you will take yourself out of your intuitive mode immediately. There will be plenty of time to apply logic later on. You will most certainly know what it feels like if you slip into analysing mode, so if you find yourself judging or interpreting just stop. Stop trying to make sense of it, for a few moments at least.

These exercises may seem challenging at first, especially if you are not used to becoming still enough to connect with your own inner dialogues but at the end of the day there are no tests to pass and no one is going to judge you on your performance. In fact you cannot fail, so be bold and give them a go.

RELAXED BREATHING TO QUIETEN THE MIND

This simple exercise need only take a few minutes and it is a great way to help you enter a more deeply relaxed and calm state of mind. It is from this quietness of mind that your most profound and valuable insights will emerge. Consider taking a few minutes to run through this exercise as a prelude to the other exercises that follow, or indeed at any time you feel the need to relax. Taking the time to quieten down enough to begin to appreciate your deeper connections also has many health benefits in itself.

Focusing your awareness on your breath is one of the best practices to help you get into the ideal state of mind for raising your awareness and for giving yourself powerful self-suggestions for change. Your breath is always there for you as an object of focus and concentration. It has a constant rhythmical cycle and it is probably one of the simplest and most rewarding meditation practices you will ever learn.

The easiest way to begin this practice is to find a time where you have ten minutes or so free, choose somewhere that you can be comfortable and relatively undisturbed and begin by making yourself comfortable either sitting or lying down. You may also like to close your eyes to help you shut out the visual distractions of the room.

Then, simply watch your breath come and go.

Become aware of your breath coming in through your nose and flowing down and into your lungs. Then watch that same process in reverse as your breath flows out again, watching in your imagination as your breath leaves your lungs, flowing out through your mouth, and out through your nose.

Continue this level of simple observation of your breath on the next cycle and the next after that.

Let this process of gentle observation continue for the next five to ten minutes, or for as long as feels comfortable for you. Observe what else is going on in your mind as you let your thoughts come and go without comment or judgment. You may well find that you cannot concentrate for more than perhaps 20 or 30 seconds at a time, before your mind starts to wander. This is normal to begin with.

It takes a while to get used to this level of stillness. As soon as you notice your mind wandering, just bring your attention back to watching your breath flowing in and out of your body. As you become more experienced with this, you may also want to place your attention on the feelings of your chest rising and falling as you breathe. Don't try to alter your breath in any way, just observe it flowing in and flowing out. Some people also like to add a colour to the breath as it flows in and out. Be spontaneous with this and just observe what happens naturally.

With practice you will find that you can go for 5 to 10 minutes at a time, without becoming too distracted. You may even notice your breathing becomes much slower and your thoughts quieter.

This is the ideal state from which to give yourself positive suggestions for change or to use as a prelude to the other exercises in this book. So keep practicing, even just a few minutes a couple of times a day will bring you real results.

HOW TO DISCOVER WHAT THE OTHER 90% OF YOUR BRAIN THINKS

Have you ever been aware that sometimes you seem to sabotage your own best interests? Or perhaps you have been trying really hard to achieve a goal but without much success. When this is the case there is often an inner 'part' or aspect of you, such as your inner child or adolescent that is still holding onto a negative belief that you acquired at some point in your past and which is now holding you back.

Finding out what your subconscious mind really thinks is often the key to moving forward, but getting good quality, reliable information from the 'back of your mind' into your conscious awareness, where you can recognise it and if needed do something about it, isn't always easy.

So let me tell you about a very simple technique you might like to try on your own to help you access your intuition and uncover some of your subconscious beliefs. It's called non-dominant hand writing. It's a form of journaling and a technique that is often used by artists and writers to help uncover limiting beliefs and release their creative abilities. You can use it too, to discover what might be getting in the way of improving your wellbeing.

This technique simply involves writing down a probing question with your dominant hand (the one you usually write with) and then putting your pen into the other hand, as you give 'permission' to your unconscious mind to provide the answer using your non-dominant hand. Don't worry about being neat, no one is going to judge you and no one need ever see what you have written.

This amazing technique can help you discover if the other 90% of your mind (the unconscious mind) is in agreement and harmony with the surface 10% of your conscious awareness. It can take courage to complete this exercise and work with the results, so start gently. It may be just a key word that comes to mind at first or you may find yourself writing a few sentences. Either way, the more harmony and understanding there can be between your conscious and unconscious beliefs the happier and more successful you are likely to be.

For example, let me tell you about a client I worked with recently called Ben.

BEN'S STORY

Ben was a young sales executive who was suffering from anxiety and high stress levels. His energy was continually low and he was beginning to feel 'out of tune' with his work. It was obvious that some 'inner part of him' was blocking his success but he wasn't consciously aware of the reason why. When he tried this exercise, he used his dominant hand to write down the question, "Dear younger me, what are you afraid of?"

Using his non-dominant hand to respond, he wrote down the words, "it's not safe" and from this came the memory that as a very young child he was always warned that it was not safe to talk to strangers. Good advice when you are only five years old, but as an adult this old unconscious belief was sabotaging his professional success as well as his mental and emotional wellbeing.

So if you are feeling blocked, fearful or stuck in any aspect of your life, try this simple exercise, you may be surprised at what you discover about yourself. After all, once you become aware of the beliefs held in your unconscious mind you can then consciously choose if you want to do something about them.

AUTOMATIC WRITING

Here is a similar exercise that you might like to try, especially if you are keeping a journal or log of your progress.

Begin by writing a sentence or two that encapsulates the challenge you are now facing. Then write in just one short sentence a question that summarise your concern. Make this question open ended, so that it cannot just be answered by yes or no. For example, rather than asking, should I be focusing on X or Y, ask something like, "what is the single most important thing I can do to improve my wellbeing"?

Next allow yourself to become quiet and still for a few moments, perhaps using the relaxed breathing exercise at the beginning of this chapter to help you enter a more calm and focused state of mind.

Now from that place of quietness, ask your question with the sincere intention of gaining the most truthful answer. Be willing to wait quietly whilst you just observe the thoughts and impressions that come along. The answers may come in the form of an image, symbol, a body sensation or a simple inner dialogue about what you need to do next.

Begin to write down any thoughts or impressions that come to you, even if it feels as though you are making it up.

If you feel blocked while you are doing this then close your eyes, take some deep breaths and try writing with your eyes closed to shut out the visual distractions of the room. It doesn't matter what your handwriting looks like. You may even like to try writing a few words with your non-dominant hand as this gives you a better link into the right side of your brain and to the information stored in the subconscious part of your mind.

Now review what you have written. What is your intuition telling you on this subject?

What action steps could you take to follow up on this information?

YOUR INNER BOARD OF HEALTH DIRECTORS

This exercise makes use of the fact that we all have inner 'parts' or aspects of ourselves that contribute to making us who we are overall. This can be very helpful to know because you can then use your imagination to engage with each part to ask it to help you achieve a particular task. I like to call this exercise your 'Inner Board of Health Directors', though you are free to change the metaphor if you wish. For example, if you don't like the idea of a board room meeting, change it to having a coffee morning with invited friends, or a simple group discussion. Hypnotherapists, NLP practitioners and coaches make regular use of this technique in their work and you can benefit too with this simple introductory exercise below.

To begin, imagine that you are the chairperson and you have a 6 member board of health directors. You and your board members meet around a conference table with 7 chairs. Your board members can be people who influence your life, people whose advice you admire, your mentor, a very close friend, someone famous or some completely mythical or unknown people.

Next, assign each of these board members names and functions, such as your nutritional advisor, your inner physician, personal trainer and so on.

All of these board members are present with one purpose only and that is to assist you in achieving your goal, in finding the solution, or in taking the best possible course of action and they all bring an extraordinary level of expertise to the table.

What will you ask of them, and what advice and feedback could they provide to assist you in fulfilling your outcome?

Use the following diagram to create a mind-map of possible solutions or just make notes beside each director's space.

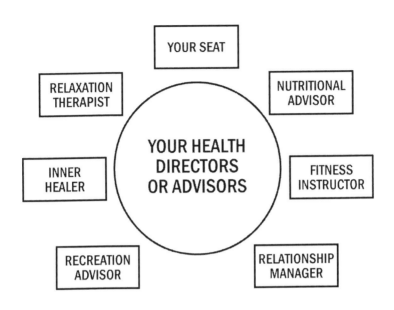

DOORWAYS TO DECISIONS

In this simple exercise you will be using the symbol of a doorway to help you gain more information about the relative value of two or more options that you have to choose from.

To begin bring to mind a choice or decision that you are having difficulty making. Define the situation clearly and think of two or three possible solutions.

Spend a few moments taking yourself to a place of mental quietness and close your eyes. Then visualise yourself in front of a door and know that this door represents your first choice or possible solution. Approach the door and notice what it is made of, how solid or strong is it? Is it locked, or easy to open? Take in as much information as you can about the qualities of this door.

Repeat this exercise with your second option as well.

Now how do the doors compare? Which one was the easiest to open and the most appealing to stand in front of? This is an excellent way for your intuition to speak to you about possible solutions, or just to give you more information about each of your choices.

You might also like to try adding a further door to represent a solution or choice you have not yet thought of.

Have fun with this simple metaphor, it is a great way of gaining extra information about a person, opportunity or thing. If you like you can also change the symbol perhaps to a tree, or a house, or a car. Any symbol will do but my advice is to keep it simple and have fun with this exercise, it is after all just a way of creating a bridge of awareness from your unconscious to your conscious mind, so that you can be better informed about the decisions ahead of you.

Once you have practiced this a couple of times you will find it a quick and easy way to use your intuition to help enhance your decision making process. Try it out on some simple choices first, for example; if you are taking any nutritional supplements you might like to ask which brands offer you the highest quality, then when you have had some practice consider using this technique as an extra resource for larger decisions such as who might be the best practitioner to help you with a particular problem.

CHAPTER SIXTEEN

THE CALL OF INTUITION

"One of the unfortunate things about our education system is that we do not teach students how to avail themselves of their subconscious capabilities."

BILL LEAR, AMERICAN INVENTOR

Many geniuses from Mozart to Einstein owe their discoveries to dreams, synchronicities or flashes of intuitive insight. Often these individuals would never have achieved their breakthroughs with logic alone and this 'non-linear intelligence' as it is sometimes called also holds great possibilities for you too once you know how to use it. I have included a chapter on it here because I believe that using your intuition can give you some really precious insights into your health and wellbeing.

It is often referred to as having a hunch, or a gut feeling about something, but whatever you chose to call it, it is that quality of direct and immediate knowledge that tells you what you need to know, when you need to know it. In other words your intuition can help to connect you with a greater knowledge than is available to your conscious mind alone. It connects you with that part of yourself that has an overview of your life and which always has your best interest at heart. Just like any other skill the more you practice the more proficient you become.

I believe that enjoying a higher level of wellness involves creating balance and wellbeing in all areas of your life and information gained from your hunches or gut instincts can be a valuable addition to enhance your normal logical thought processes. I've worked with many people over the years who have been surprised at the quality of information that can come through in this way. It has certainly helped me whenever I have felt stuck, or blocked, or simply undecided as to which way to go. So I would like to share some of my discoveries with you in the hope that you will find them interesting and decide it is worthwhile to develop your sixth sense too.

To use your intuition is a very natural thing to do. You don't need any special skills to do it, just a genuine desire to get results and the commitment to practice with focused attention. One of the main reasons why it can be such a valuable asset is that it gives you a resource that provides an additional level of information that does not come from the logical, analytical or rational side of your mind alone. Perhaps you have already had the experience of having a gut feeling about something where you suddenly know something that your conscious mind was unaware of. The trick is to be able to summon this information on demand, consciously and on purpose. It is a natural skill that we all possess, but like any other kind of skill, it gets better with the right kind of practice.

Using your 'sixth sense' is very definitely a skill that can be learnt and it can be a valuable tool in helping you to make wise and healthy choices, or to simply become more aware of the messages your body may be trying to give you about what it needs.

The first thing you need to be able to do is to identify and distinguish your genuine insights from the background noise of fear, desires, imaginings and normal mental chatter. Next you need to learn to trust and follow your hunches. Listening to the heart as some people describe it is a key to getting more information. Your intuitive guidance system is sensitive and if its messages are not being appreciated, they will soon diminish in frequency. On the other hand with the right type of cultivation they will increase in both frequency and accuracy so that you can come to trust and rely on this inner intelligence.

So how do you go about developing your intuition? There is no mystical secret here just basic information and lots of practice. Most of all though you need to pay attention to it, everyone can do it, the difference is that some people listen to this subtle information and act upon it whilst others discount it.

A sign in Albert Einstein's office is rumoured to have read:

"Not everything that can be counted counts, and not everything that counts can be counted."

HOW DOES YOUR INTUTION SPEAK TO YOU?
Your intuition works rather like a radio signal which sweeps through the frequencies looking for your favourite radio station and that momentary signal as you cross through the stations reflects just how fast your sixth sense works. It can take care and experience to become skilled in the deciphering of those signals but when you get going it is fun, fast and very accurate.

These hunches when they come can attract your attention in many different ways. For some people it is more of an emotional response, a 'gut' reaction that tells you if something is fundamentally good or bad, for others it may be a mixture of mental images or symbols that can appear in your imagination or dreams and for yet others it may even be a physical sensation or an external synchronicity or coincidence.

Think about this for yourself. How do your 'hunches' most frequently get your attention? Is it a physical sensation, an inner knowing, a change in your energy, what is it? In general the sooner you start noticing how your intuition attracts your attention the more quickly you will be able to recognise it when it comes.

OBSTACLES AND PITFALLS

Another important point is to become aware of some of the obstacles that might be blocking you from becoming more insightful about your health. For most people it is their logical mind that turns out to be the biggest block of all because it usually wants to seek proof of the validity of the information before accepting it and of course your intuition just doesn't work that way.

So don't try to second guess what your instinct might be telling you, or let your intellect, fears or desires slip in with some unhelpful comment, or additional information. Aim to immediately acknowledge any information that you get in response to your questions without judgement, or tying to work it out.

For many people setting expectations that are too high is also a cause of disappointment and failure. The goal in the beginning is simply to train yourself to become more aware of the more subtle information your body is giving you about your needs. Be patient with yourself and as you practice you will get more and more confident that the information you are picking up on is reliable and valid.

If you tried out some of the exercises in the last chapter such as *Your Inner Board of Health Directors*, or *Doorways to Decisions*, then you will already be familiar with the importance of symbols in helping you to interpret your hunches. Don't worry about trying to find a literal interpretation of these symbols, just accept that the language of symbols and metaphors is part of the way your intuition speaks to you on a daily basis. If you haven't tried those exercises yet I suggest you bookmark them for another time when you can put them to the test. Make sure that in the beginning you try them out on the situations, people or things that you can assess with your logical mind too, so that you can begin to develop some trust and confidence in the process.

Last but not least you need to keep asking the next question. Initially it is tempting to be so pleased with any response you get to your first question that you stop there. Don't, keep asking. Get into the habit of asking for further information, perhaps from a different perspective and then ask for a clear interpretation of any information that you pick up on.

KAREN'S STORY

Let me share Karen's story with you to help you appreciate just how important your hunches can be.

Karen was about three quarters of the way through her pregnancy when I met her. She was thoroughly enjoying being pregnant and the focus of our coaching together was on helping her make the transition to becoming a working mother as smooth as possible. Her greatest challenge was on letting go of her role at work and keeping her stress levels under control. As her pregnancy progressed she realised that if she didn't start to delegate her workload and agree an action plan for her return then she would soon find these decisions taken out of her hands. So much of our coaching was focused around planning an acceptable work/life balance.

One day as she was getting ready for work she started to get a strong 'gut-feeling' that all might not be well with her pregnancy. Her words were that this felt like, "an urgency to get help", with a nervous feeling in her stomach that just wasn't logical. Karen was already very good at paying attention to her gut feelings so although there was no obvious reason to do so she decided to work from home that day. She was absolutely fine all morning but later on that afternoon she went into premature labour and was admitted to hospital.

In the end both she and her baby were fine, but by listening to her intuition that day she gave herself the very best chance of being prepared for what was to come.

Over the years I've come across many people who have really benefitted by listening to their hunches. You can use it in a hundred different ways to help you make the healthiest choices. You can even use it for the simple little things like helping you to pick the freshest and best quality food in the marketplace. It's all helpful.

SOME HELPFUL TIPS:
Finally let me offer you my top ten tips that I have come to value over the years to help you build you intuitive awareness of how you can improve your wellbeing.

1. Quieten down. Noise, especially a noisy mind makes it impossible to listen to what your sixth sense is telling you. Find some time each day to be quiet with your thoughts.

2. Stay focused and in the present with your attention directed outward on the task in hand. Aim to have a period of quiet reflection or meditation each day, or schedule an appointment with yourself in your diary to give yourself some quiet and undisturbed time for reflection.

3. Keep your stress levels down. When you are stressed you are not paying attention to much else and the speed and subtly of your inner hunches can easily be lost or overridden.

4. Learn to recognise how your intuition 'speaks' to you. How does it most frequently attract your attention? With fleeting images, by interrupting your mental chatter with an unexpected thought, or perhaps by some physical sensation.

5. Be prepared to follow through. The information you gain will be useless unless you act on it.

6. Make a note of these subtle impressions as soon as you can after receiving them. Your intuition is held in your short term memory and can easily be forgotten, so record your impressions accurately as soon as you receive them, making sure that you don't add anything from your logical thought processes.

7. Realise that your 'sixth-sense' will always come to you via your own filters of beliefs, prejudices and cultural assumptions. Being aware of this will help as much information get through as possible.

8. If you have a strong personal need be aware that it is also likely to colour the information you receive.

9. Try to tie in your 'gut-reactions' with other forms of knowledge. Several indicators together are much stronger than one alone.

10. Practice acting on your gut feelings to build your sense of confidence in your own abilities. Use it or lose it as the saying goes.

ACTIVITY: ASKING YOUR INTUITION

If you were to quieten down enough to ask your intuition right now if there is anything you should either start doing or stop doing to help improve your wellbeing, what would your answers be?

CHAPTER SEVENTEEN

POSITIVE PERSONAL ENERGY AND WHY YOU SHOULD CARE ABOUT IT

"There is a vitality, a life force, an energy,
a quickening, that is translated through you
into action, and because there is only one of you
in all time, this expression is unique."
MARTHA GRAHAM, AMERICAN DANCE TEACHER AND CHOREOGRAPHER 1894-1991

DISCOVERING YOUR VITALITY

By now you will probably have had time to think a great deal about the words health and wellness and what they might mean to you but now I would also like you to think about another concept; your vitality. Many people are familiar with the concept of 'vitality', but very few understand exactly what it is.

For some people vibrancy and vitality means having more stamina and the ability to maintain a high pressure lifestyle, to others it may simply mean enjoying good health and a greater degree of inner contentment.

My own interpretation is simply that our vitality is a measure of the quantity and quality of the life force energy that we have available to us. Having a strong vitality allows you to respond to the world around you with ease and to be able to adapt and change without undue stress. But these are just my thoughts, what is far more important is what the concept of vitality means to you.

What words or images come to mind when you consider your own vitality?

Are there any more words you would like to add for the future?

Perhaps you have noticed how many food products, herbal and nutritional supplements make a play on this word in their marketing campaigns, all in an attempt to align their product with something that is essential to life. In reality of course the best that most of these products can do is to stimulate your vitality on a short term basis. Clearly this is not the route to achieving a high level of wellness that is both durable and sustainable over time.

The good news however is that we all have the potential to enhance our vitality, to be even happier, healthier and stronger. Becoming more conscious of the quality of your vital energy on a day to day basis is a great way to begin.

ARE YOU ENERGY CONSCIOUS?

Do you ever end up feeling drained at the end of the day, or perhaps you are always playing catch up with yourself, never feeling that you quite have enough energy to do everything that actually needs to be done? These are common feelings and if your 'energy account' remains in the red, or unbalanced, then the long term result can be exhaustion and ultimately a level of stress that is difficult to relieve. So what can you do about this?

One answer is to become more energy conscious, to become aware of how your energy is flowing, where you may be wasting it, blocking it, or letting it leak away. Then of course you need to discover what you can do about it.

Our energy, like our time, is an incredibly precious resource, and maintaining its flow is fundamental to good health. Yet however efficiently we may seem to manage it, there is still no guarantee that we will have enough to do all that we might like to do and for many people it is often a lack of energy rather than a lack of time that is the greater challenge. But just like time, and money, your energy levels can be managed too. With just a little forethought and a commitment to take action the results can be astounding and can take you a long way along the path of greater wellness.

One of the keys to becoming more energy conscious is to start noticing how you are spending your energy. For example, you may start to become more aware of who, or what leaves you feeling drained or depleted, what times of day you naturally feel the most energized or lethargic, or how the company of different people affects you. For some people even the weather makes a difference. Of course, it is equally important to pay attention to what energises you too. Think about this for a moment, what times of day, or activities, or environments tend to uplift and replenish you if you are feeling a bit low?

ACTIVITY: YOUR ENERGY WHEEL
It can often help to 'draw out' what you are thinking by creating a simple picture that can be interpreted at a glance. The *Wheel of Wellness* exercise at the

147

beginning of this book is a good example and you can use exactly the same technique to draw yourself an energy wheel too.

In this exercise the outer edge of your wheel or pie chart represents a strong and vibrant flow of energy, with a maximum score of ten, with the centre carrying a score of naught, reflecting feelings of complete exhaustion or depletion.

Now in the same way as you have done before divide this 'wheel' into six or eight segments to reflect your energy levels in various aspects of your life, for example; your primary relationships, your job, or quality of sleep. Give an appropriate label to each of these segments and then allow yourself a few minutes of quiet reflection to assess the quality of your energy in each area.

Give each spoke of your wheel a number which you mark on your circle somewhere between 1 and 10 and then join up each segment to create a new outline. Is the outline of your energy wheel bumpy or smooth? Does it reflect good quality energy and a high level of vitality in some areas of your life but not others?

What does this picture of your energy tell you about the way you spend and replenish your energy that you didn't really appreciate before?

This is really precious information because as you become more energy conscious you can also begin to develop strategies to increase your vitality in times of challenge or stress, or deliberately factor some activities into your day that you know will boost your energy. Perhaps a brisk walk, listening to some lively music, having a good laugh, or taking a power nap. Knowing what works best for you is important, but far more important is that you actually use this information for your own benefit each and every day.

We are all energised by different things, so start noticing where your life really gives you energy, where you are running in neutral, or heading towards depletion. Now, with that new information, take a moment to be your own coach and ask yourself:

"What health enhancing steps could I take to help strengthen my vitality and feel more energised?"

Your energy wheel will give you a clue to the answer here. Pick an area where your score was low and consider if there is something that you could either start doing, or stop doing that would give you real and measurable improvements over time.

I'm not talking about temporary energy boosters such as a strong cup of coffee, as these are usually only short term interventions, often at the expense of your overall energy store. Making a withdrawal on your energy account by using stimulants can mean that the long term result can be even greater fatigue, especially if you don't also take steps to allow yourself to recover and replenish your energy.

Think about this, if there was just one thing that you could do that would make a real difference to your vibrancy and quality of energy on a daily basis, what would it be?

Here are just a few examples for you to consider:

- Break out of your routines occasionally and schedule some 'me' time, to do something different and fun.

- Tidy up the space around you. The less clutter you have to wade though, the more energy you will have to devote to other things.

- Eat small regular meals, to help you maintain a constant supply of energy throughout the day.

- Get an energy boost by trying something new and adding different experiences to your day, or give your senses a treat by indulging in some new aromas, tastes or vibrant colours.

- Breathe deeply. Stop occasionally to take five extra full deep breaths, to help increase your alertness.

- Get a good night's sleep, so that your body has its best chance to repair, restore and rejuvenate.

- Last but not least, ask yourself if you would be really willing to make that change and do what it takes to enjoy even greater vibrancy and vitality?

If your energy levels are already really good, or if you don't feel sufficiently motivated to change at this point, just be grateful for any insights you may have received from this simple exercise and move on.

If on the other hand your answer is a resounding 'yes', then as soon as you have finished reading this page, go and get yourself a pen and paper and write down your commitment to take action.

The quality of your daily energy is a really important factor in your overall wellbeing. So if you would like a little bit more vibrancy and sparkle in your life consider setting aside a few minutes each day to review your personal energy account. You won't regret it.

WATCH OUT FOR ENERGY VAMPIRES!

As well as including more things that sustain a healthy energy level in your day, you may also need to take steps to watch out for those people or things that drain your energy too. People who do this to you are often labelled as energy vampires and they come in all shapes and sizes but here are a few tips to help you recognise them.

- **The drama queen** – these people always make a big deal out of nothing and can leave you feeling tired and listless.

- **The intruder** – anyone who ignores your personal boundaries and privacy probably doesn't care very much about you.

- **The blamer** – these people are seldom willing to take responsibility for themselves. So watch out, they will be looking for someone to blame.

- **The complainer** – they constantly seem to be complaining about their partners, jobs, illnesses and just about anything else they can get you to listen to.

- **The critic** – these people seldom have anything good to say, either about you or anything else.

CHAPTER EIGHTEEN

MIND OVER MATTER AND MENTAL REHEARSAL

"It is madness to only prepare yourself physically and to leave your mental frame of mind to chance. The difference that makes the difference is learning how to feel strong in your mind as well as your body. Every athlete should understand that you don't have to have a gold medal around your neck to feel like a champion."
ROGER BLACK M.B.E, OLYMPIC SILVER MEDALLIST

FAKE IT TILL YOU MAKE IT

Athletes do it and top performers wouldn't be without it, I am of course talking about using the power of your mind to help you achieve success. The fact is that when your mental images are accompanied by strong emotions they form the blueprints of your reality. Of course this is absolutely nothing new, in fact the simple steps of using desire, imagination and expectancy to help you achieve success have been known since ancient times but what is so exciting is that they are now also being upheld by the latest scientific discoveries, especially within the field of quantum physics.

Once you know what you want then the next logical step in the process of coaching yourself is to draw up an action plan to go out and get it but I would like to suggest another step along the way and that is to 'pretend' that you already have it. Fake it till you make it the saying goes. Pretending that you already have what you want is not a new idea, nor is it just another crazy new age strategy which leaves you with your head in the clouds. It has real value because when you pretend that you already have the qualities of the thing that you want, you begin to harness the conscious direction of your thoughts towards actually achieving it.

By mentally rehearsing your success you are creating an inspiring vision of the future to help increase your readiness for change. It helps to build up the motivation you need to keep focused on your goals and shows you how to focus on an all together bigger, brighter and bolder vision of yourself.

One of the truly fascinating things about mental rehearsal is that it is the subject of a great deal of research at the moment which shows that by actively rehearsing an outcome in your mind you are actually creating the same neural patterns and pathways in your brain as by doing the real thing. Perhaps the best news of all though is that these same techniques that are used by athletes the world over can actually be used by you too, to help improve your performance, or increase your alignment with your goals.

HOW MENTAL REHEARSAL WORKS

It's a fascinating fact but your brain cannot always tell the difference between what is real and imagined and current research suggests that this strange phenomenon can be invaluable when it comes to improving your outcomes, including helping you to heal or improve your wellbeing. Put simply, your body responds to your thoughts, so what you pay attention to really matters. If you stop to think about this for a moment you will find many examples in your everyday life, take blushing for example, or salivating at the thought of a tasty snack, or even sexual arousal. They are all physical responses in the body that have been stimulated by thoughts and images in your mind.

In fact your subconscious mind sees to it that you automatically act according to the thoughts and images you hold in your subconscious database. For example, when you say, "that's easy for me," you find it easy and of course the opposite is true too, if you believe that something is going to be difficult or hard for you then it probably will be.

Just about everyone can use imagery successfully to bring about some positive changes in their life. You can do it too even if you don't think of yourself as being particularly visual. Some people naturally prefer to get a sense of what can be heard or felt rather than what can be seen and that will work too as long as what you are experiencing connects you directly to that concept of your potential. In essence if you can daydream, you can do it. Perhaps you have already heard of the saying 'a picture is worth a thousand words'? Well that has never been more true than with the use of guided imagery and mental rehearsal, as the mental images of success that you create act as a bridge between the conscious and unconscious parts of your mind and help to bring about real change.

IT'S NOT JUST ABOUT DAYDREAMING

But let me also offer a word of caution here not to confuse true mental rehearsal with the techniques of guided imagery or visualisation. Technically when you rehearse a future outcome you should be looking out through your own eyes as if you were actually an actor in your own movie, whereas guided imagery or visualisation techniques are more akin to active daydreaming where you are looking at yourself as if you were on a mental screen of some sort, observing the whole situation rather than experiencing it directly.

Being in such a strongly associated state makes this a much more powerful technique than simply visualising what you want but for the purposes of this book I believe both of these techniques have tremendous value as coaching tools as both can help inspire and motivate you towards greater wellness.

GETTING THE MOST FROM GUIDED IMAGERY

The first step to successfully coaching yourself is to build up your desire for what you want. Your desires are the motivating force that push you towards your goals and having a strong passion for something means that your mind is also actively involved in searching for solutions for you.

Once you are really clear about what you want your new outcome to be, you need to add as much vivid detail to that picture of success as you can. This helps your subconscious mind understand clearly what it is that you want to achieve. Mental rehearsal, visualisation and guided imagery techniques are all really useful to use alongside coaching and they all use images as a form of 'language' to appeal to that part of your brain that can 'communicate' with your body to help bring about changes or achievements. Of them all, guided imagery is probably the easiest to practice on your own and I have included a short guide here, by way of example, to help get you started.

Finally, my advice is to keep it simple. Don't try and do too much on your first session. Just pick one aspect of what it is that you want to achieve. This will help make your results more measurable and give you the confidence to carry on.

Before moving on let me mention a couple of concerns that are often raised about these techniques. Firstly, some people think that all this inner reflection about your ideal state is encouraging you to live in fantasy land but really this is not the case at all. All that I am suggesting here is that you engage your active imagination in a few moments of vivid imagery each day to give your subconscious mind the clear message that you intend to change. Secondly, some people worry that because they find it difficult to see pictures in their mind that these techniques won't work. But they will work just as long as you can create a vivid sensory impression of your success using any of your senses and if you can also add the feelings of achievement then so much the better.

Even if you are not sure that these techniques can work for you I would encourage you to have a go, just actively daydreaming a little bit more about having what you want, or falling asleep at night imagining yourself enjoying your new success will all be helpful.

THE EXPERIMENT
This simple guided imagery exercise that I have called *'The Experiment'* can be used as a visualisation technique by looking at yourself as if you were playing

a part in your own mental movie, or as a mental rehearsal technique by imagining yourself actually stepping into that image of the 'future you' and looking out through your own eyes rather than looking on.

In a moment I'm going to invite you to take a sneak peak at what the healthier and happier you might be like. I'm going to invite you to imagine that future part of you that has already been successful; a future part that already exists just a short distance into the future from now.

Imagine you are reading this rather like a bed time story and let my words encourage your imagination to show you your potential.

Make yourself comfortable now and become aware of your breathing for a moment as you begin to relax and enter a quieter and more focused state of awareness. Let the focus of your awareness be inside your imagination, just for a little while.

And in your imagination, become aware that you have the opportunity to take part in a fascinating experiment to find out what the future you might be like... and like most experiments this one requires that you sign a form giving your consent... so become aware of this form now in your mind's eye...

And as you imagine this contract in front of you, get a sense of what the words on the page may say... perhaps there are certain things that you need to agree to start... or stop doing... if this trial is to be successful... after all a contract should always be read extremely carefully before you sign it and give your consent to change...

158

Because if this experiment works... Something wonderful and new and different will happen and I want to be sure that you have really agreed to this.

So if and only if you are ready, sign that form now giving your subconscious mind your consent to go in search of those positive changes for you.

And although this is just your own personal experiment... It is important for you to know that many other people have gone before you and their results have been excellent... I mention this because the chances are that you will get really good results too.

Get a sense of that future version of you now... a future you that is willing to try out new ways of thinking and new ways of doing things... and I wonder what ideas you will try out first on your way to reaching your milestone or achieving your goal... allow these images to become as vivid and bright as possible... give yourself a few moments to play around with those images...

Now of course as with any experiment it can take time for all the results to be published, or evident for other people to see... but because they are your results you can have a sneak preview... A glimpse ahead of time... to look at the results of your new beliefs or your new choices.

So take a look at those results now by running a mental movie in your imagination as you enjoy those new choices that you finally decided upon

...for standing in front of you now is the you that has already made the best choices... has got the best results... notice how this future version of you had to change to be successful... perhaps letting go of some

old beliefs... or by doing new things... and I wonder which aspects of these changes you will find the most surprising and the most pleasing?

Allow yourself a little more time to enjoy this mental movie... turning up the brightness... the colour... the sound... rewinding or pausing that flow of images if you would like to... they are your images and you are free to enjoy them in any way you wish.

And even though it may take a little time for those final results to be published in the real world, that doesn't matter because you have already had a glimpse of what is to come and you know that this experiment has already been successful.

And the truly amazing thing is that this successful you already exists as a potential just a little way into the future from now... and if that future you could reach back through time to give your present self some advice... what would that advice be?

You may even like to imagine stepping into that image of yourself for a moment, looking out through your own eyes at the changes that have occurred... what do you see and hear that tells you... you have already been successful? How do you feel?

And one of the greatest benefits of this experiment is that you don't have to keep these changes if you really don't like them. Yet with your permission your subconscious mind will continue this work on your behalf... without any conscious effort on your part at all... you might even like to give your subconscious mind your permission to continue to make these changes on your behalf whilst you sleep at night... knowing that you can revisit these results as often as you wish to see just how well those changes are progressing.

Allow yourself a little longer to enjoy these scenes... and then when you are ready gently return your awareness fully and completely back into the present moment.

Returning with all the learning you need from this experience to help you take the next step and the then the step after that on your journey to better health.

Bringing your attention fully back to normal alert awareness... bringing back with you all the new understandings this experience has given you... as you become vividly aware of what is in the room around you now so that you can safely carry on with your day.

ACTIVITY: CREATE YOUR OWN MENTAL MOVIE

Now think of something about yourself that you would like to improve on and practice creating your own short mental movie in which you have achieved these improvements.

For example, many people like to rehearse reaching one of their milestones on the way to greater goal achievement.

Make this mental movie as vivid and real as you can. Do you look, feel, or think differently now that you have achieved this milestone? Perhaps you can hear other people congratulating you, or perhaps something has changed about your physical appearance that you can see. Take your time to imagine yourself in the most vivid detail that you can. Then ask what you could do in the present to help move yourself towards that future success.

GETTING RESULTS

I'm often asked how long it will take to get results with these techniques and the answer really depends on many factors such as the extent to which you need or want to change and how well you can maintain a state of focused attention on your new outcomes.

At first you will probably find that you can only hold these images for a couple of seconds at a time. Don't worry most of us aren't really used to holding our attention still for very long but even a few seconds placed with focused intent on your success and then repeated regularly throughout the day will be helpful.

With practice you will probably find that you can hold your attention on your 'rehearsal' for much longer, say up to 20-30 seconds at a time which will be much more effective. You could also help yourself by choosing to dream of your success as you naturally fall asleep at bedtime, or perhaps make yourself a simple recording by adapting the suggestions I've given you here, or even making up some of your own. Just remember to make it entirely personal to you and as specific as you can.

In general terms the more often and the more clearly that you can focus your attention on the vivid images of yourself being healthy and well, then the better your results will be.

CHAPTER NINETEEN

WHAT'S NEXT?

"Our deepest fear is not that we are inadequate. Our deepest fear is that we are powerful beyond measure. It is our light, not our darkness, that most frightens us. We ask ourselves, who am I to be brilliant, gorgeous, talented and fabulous? Actually, who are you not to be?"
MARIANNE WILLIAMSON, AMERICAN AUTHOR AND LECTURER 1952

WHAT'S LOVE GOT TO DO WITH IT?

What's love got to do with coaching yourself to better health?

Well actually quite a lot. Firstly having just a little bit more love for yourself can make a huge difference when it comes to being able to summon up enough energy to actually make a change. And then there is the love you have for your family and friends, how will your willingness to change, or perhaps your decision to stay the same affect your ability to show your love and care for the people closest to you?

I believe that ultimately we are all connected and we all need to give and receive love to be truly healthy. Experiencing love for ourselves and others is fundamental to living a life of high quality wellness and the extent to which you are able to love and care for yourself will be felt not only by your family but by the wider community around you too.

Look back to your answers in the *Chain of Consequences* activity and consider what might happen if you don't have enough self-love to keep yourself in the best of health. How will that decision radiate out into your family and wider community?

Of course the opposite of love is fear and fear is probably one of the strongest forces that will hold you back. But recognising how that affects you isn't always that easy. Here are just a few of the more commonly held fear-based beliefs that can hold you back. Perhaps you can recognise some aspects of yourself here, or maybe add some more examples of your own.

FEAR OF FAILURE

This is probably top of the list for most people. Think about it, how often have you simply decided not to even try in case you failed? I can think of lots of my own examples and I'm sure that you could come up with a few examples of your own too. Yet to avoid the risk of failure is also to avoid the opportunity to learn and without learning it becomes much harder to grow and progress.

FEAR OF SUCCESS

This tends to be quite a bit harder to spot and even harder to admit to but it can still cut across your will to succeed, so it's well worth being aware of. Success usually brings some measure of change along with it and the challenge of newness and the unknown can be very scary. Of course this may not apply to you, especially if all you want to do is to make some small adjustments to your wellbeing but if you are hoping to make changes that other people will notice too, then be aware that there may be a part of you that might just be afraid of your potential success.

FEAR OF BEING JUDGED, OR OF LOSING THE LOVE OF SOMEONE SPECIAL

It may sound obvious but change always brings with it new consequences, not all of which may be entirely welcome. Be aware that your new choices may well put the spotlight on the more unhealthy activities of your friends, family or colleagues which may be uncomfortable for them. They may even try to sabotage your success.

For example, if you lose a significant amount of weight this might set up resistance amongst other family members who may also feel pressurised to follow your example. The trick here is to be aware of these potential consequences well ahead of time so that you can plan to mitigate them. Being consciously aware of any potential judgements that may be coming your way will be a great help when it comes to working through them. So be sensitive about this and respect the comfort zones of the people around you as you move forward yourself. One day they may well see you as a role model, so don't take your eye off your goal.

WHAT HAVE YOU LEARNT SO FAR?

Any teacher will tell you that it is a good thing to stop and review your progress from time to time and the same applies to coaching yourself too. So let me ask you a few important questions.

- Firstly what have you learnt so far from this book that will help you improve your health and wellbeing?

- And given what you have learnt, what is the next thing that you could do to either improve a specific aspect of your health or enhance your overall wellbeing?

- Would you be willing to do it?

I really want to encourage you to make your self-coaching time a priority even if that might also mean thinking about how you can make yourself more of a priority too. It needn't take long and if you can make some improvements to the quality of your life then surely it's worth it.

TIME TO CELEBRATE

By now you may already have some small achievements to celebrate, or perhaps even some major ones as you take steady focused steps towards your goal. Wherever you are in the process of change, it is of tremendous importance that you take some time to acknowledge all that you have achieved and confirm your success by celebrating the change. This doesn't have to be expensive but it does have to be meaningful.

Whatever you choose to do make sure that you hold in your mind your gratitude for what you have achieved so far. This is really important because as you do this, you are giving a strong and clear message to your subconscious mind that you have already achieved your goal, even and perhaps especially if that change is still ongoing. It reinforces your 'template' for success as well as giving you something to look forward to. Quite simply it fuels your motivation for enjoying even greater things to come and gives you the encouragement to keep going. After all, if you never allow yourself to stop and take stock of what you have achieved you will be denying yourself much of the satisfaction of achieving your goals.

So think about some of your successes so far, even the small ones and tell yourself, "well done".

ACTIVITY: CELEBRATE YOUR ACHIEVEMENTS

Make a note of how and when you would like to celebrate your achievements, however small, or large they may be. Check to make sure that the way in which you have chosen to celebrate doesn't in itself detract from your wellbeing (in other words, big boxes of chocolates don't count) and then write a date in your diary to mark the time by which you intend to be ready to celebrate your goal, or milestone.

WHAT'S NEXT?

CHAPTER TWENTY

A FINAL FEW WORDS ON COACHING YOURSELF

I hope you have been able to use some of the suggestions and activities in this book to make some valuable improvements to your wellbeing. As you will have discovered, reading this material alone will do little for you, you must take action if you really want to see results.

Before I became a professional coach I was a lecturer in nursing and midwifery, and one of my favourite quotes to encourage my students to learn comes from Florence Nightingale, one of the founders of the modern day nursing profession. It's this:

> *"I do not pretend to teach her how, I ask*
> *her to teach herself, and for this purpose*
> *I venture to give her some hints."*
> FLORENCE NIGHTINGALE 1860

Now that you have a good insight into how coaches work, perhaps you can see why I like this quote so much. Because I don't know you personally I cannot pretend to coach you. I can only ask that you coach yourself and for this purpose I too have ventured to give you some hints.

Whether you want more of something, or less of something, the bottom line is always about change and as you learn to coach yourself to better health you will be continually opening up new possibilities for yourself and at the same time learning to become very focused on your results.

For some people, generating enthusiasm and staying on track is easy. For others it can at times seem to be quite a struggle. If this has been the case for you, then you may benefit from finding a 'buddy' to co-coach with, or consider working alongside a professional for a while, until you generate the momentum you need for change.

Coaching yourself to better health doesn't mean that you have to go on this journey alone. It is perfectly alright to ask for help and support when you need it. Many people actually prefer the personal support that comes from working with a professional, so if this applies to you, choose carefully and remember to always ask for a free sample session, or at least the opportunity to ask your coach questions by phone or email to make sure that their style suits you.

One last thing; this is not a one off exercise. You need to keep at it. You need to keep asking the next question and then the question after that which will lead you in the direction of greater health.

Like anything else, with practice, this will become a habit and the day will come when it will seem natural to you to engage the help of your inner coach whenever you feel that something is lacking in your life, or when you need to raise the bar on your personal best.

As our journey together comes to an end I hope that you have been able to learn some really valuable and precious things about your potential. Perhaps you have been able to celebrate some small improvements, or even a couple of major ones. Most of all I hope that you have felt a sense of pride in your ability to take control.

It is never too late to enhance your wellbeing and coaching yourself to better health is one of the best tools you will come across to help you bring a greater vibrancy and vitality to life.

Wherever you are in this process I wish you joy on your journey.

BIBLIOGRAPHY

Arloski, Michael, *Wellness Coaching for Lasting Lifestyle Change*, Whole Person Associates 2007

Barber, Judy, *Good Question!: The Art of Asking Questions to Bring About Positive Change*, Lean Marketing Press 2005

Gee, Judee, *Intuition Awakening Your Inner Guide*, Samuel Weser 1999

Grabhorn, Lynn, *Excuse me your Life is Waiting*, Hampton Roads Publishing Co. 2000

Grant, Anthony & Greene, Jane, *Coach Yourself*, Pearson Education Limited 2004

Hamilton, David, *How Your Mind Can Heal Your Body*, Hay House 2008

Kassy, Karen Grace, *Health Intuition*, Hazelden Information & Educational Services 2000

Maltz, Maxwell, *Psycho-cybernetics*, Prentice Hall Press, 2003

McKenna, Paul, Change *Your Life in Seven Days*, Bantam Press, 2004

Prochaska, James, Norcross, John & Diclemente, Carlo, *Changing for Good*, Collins Living 2006

Seward, Brian Luke, *Health and Wellness Journal Workbook, Second Ed.*, Jones and Bartlett Publishers 2003

Whitmore, John, *Coaching for Performance*, Nicholas Brealey Publishing, 2009

Whitworth, Laura, Kimsey-House, Henry & Sandahl, Phil, *Co-Active Coaching*, Davies-Black Publishing 1998

Williamson, Marianne, *A Return to Love*, Thorsons 1996

RESOURCES

FIRST WAY FORWARD
www.firstwayforward.com

For relaxation and hypnotherapy CDs and digital downloads with ranges for adults and children which will help enhance physical, mental and emotional well being. More than fifteen titles for adults and more than twenty titles for children of all age groups, starting at 4 years of age. New recordings are being added all the time. Do visit the site and listen to extracts to help you choose the right ones for you.

FREE ACTIVITY DOWNLOADS
www.AnneLesleyMarshall.co.uk/book-offer.html

This is where you can claim your free downloads of some of the activities mentioned in this book.

KEEP THE CHANGE: WELLNESS COACHING PROGRAMME
www.Keep-The-Change.co.uk

Based on this book this wellness coaching programme is designed help you achieve your personal health goals, fulfill a lifestyle prescription, be supported through a challenging health transition, or simply to feel better about yourself.

It is ideally suited to anyone who wants, or needs, to make some improvements to their baseline level of health and includes up to six one hour telephone coaching sessions backed up by email support throughout the course.

NHS CHOICES LIVE WELL

www.nhs.uk/livewell/Pages/Livewellhub.aspx

Unbiased information on healthy living choices. Click on the tools section to check if you are a healthy weight, need to track your alcohol consumption, get fitness tips, or learn more about your health.

NOBLE-MANHATTAN COACHING

www.noble-manhattan.com

Offers accredited Life Coach Training and NLP Training programmes. Their website provides a wealth of resources and information for people who want to learn more about coaching.

THE MAYO CLINIC

www.mayoclinic.com

Award-winning medical and health information and tools for healthy living

THE INTERNATIONAL INSTITUTE OF COACHING

www.internationalinstituteofcoaching.com

The IIC (formerly the European Coaching Institute) was founded by and continues to be run by professional Coaches. As an Internationally focused organisation its aim is to promote best practice within the field of coaching.

LIKE TO KNOW MORE?

I hope you have enjoyed discovering how to coach yourself to better health but the end of the book isn't the end of the story, it's really just the beginning.

If you would like my personal support, my e-course which comes with a full 90 days of email support is a great place to start.

www.annelesleymarshall.co.uk/better-health.html

If you would like to learn more about how coaching can be used either within the workplace or a healthcare environment then have a look at my seminars listings at *www.annelesleymarshall.co.uk/Seminars.html* and if you don't see exactly what you want there give me a call and ask me to create a bespoke course proposal for you.

Whichever option you chose, enjoy the learning!

MY FREE GIFTS TO YOU

WWW.COACH-YOURSELF.CO.UK

As a coach my aim is to help you create a clear vision for your continued wellbeing and if you would like to keep in touch then please accept my invitation to visit me at www.Coach-Yourself.co.uk where you will find many resources that you can download and print out, or add to your journal.

You will also find some extra resources, not mentioned here in the book. They are my personal thank you for your support.

If you would like to work with me one to one, then I suggest you start by having a look at the various formats of coaching that I can offer you. Then request a free sample session by phone or email, so that we can both be sure that I am the best person to help. You'll find all the information you need at *www.AnneLesleyMarshall.co.uk*

I'll see you there.

Printed in Great Britain
by Amazon.co.uk, Ltd.,
Marston Gate.